Contemporary Issues in Clinical Bioethics - Medical, Ethical and Legal Perspectives

Edited by Peter Clark and Kamil Hakan Dogan

Published in London, United Kingdom

Contemporary Issues in Clinical Bioethics - Medical, Ethical and Legal Perspectives
http://dx.doi.org/10.5772/intechopen.1000428
Edited by Peter Clark and Kamil Hakan Dogan

Contributors
Ashish P. Anjankar, Borislav R. Yoshinov, Bridget Ellul, Cesar Hernandez Mier, Codrin Horea Rebeleanu, Dana Doroftei, Daniel Disandro, Ivet B. Koleva, Jennifer Garcia Ospina, Joseph Kelly, Julieta S. Gerenova, Ka-Huen Yip, Mahvish Renzu, Namrata Anjankar, Osamu Muramoto, Patricia Eugenia Diaz Montoya, Peter Clark, Radoslav R. Yoshinov, Richmond Ekhosuehi Idaeho, Salvador Ribas Ribas, Sandra Vianney Ramírez Ojeda, Sara Casati, Shrikanth Sampath, Teodora A. Asenova, Urban Vrtacnik, Vaibhav Anjankar, Wai-King Tsui, Yuk-Chiu Yip

First published in London, United Kingdom, 2024 by IntechOpen
IntechOpen is the global imprint of INTECHOPEN LIMITED, registered in England and Wales, registration number: 11086078, 5 Princes Gate Court, London, SW7 2QJ, United Kingdom

British Library Cataloguing-in-Publication Data
A catalogue record for this book is available from the British Library

Additional hard and PDF copies can be obtained from orders@intechopen.com

Contemporary Issues in Clinical Bioethics - Medical, Ethical and Legal Perspectives
Edited by Peter Clark and Kamil Hakan Dogan
p. cm.
Print ISBN 978-1-83769-715-1
Online ISBN 978-1-83769-714-4
eBook (PDF) ISBN 978-1-83769-716-8

For EU product safety concerns:
IN TECH d.o.o., Prolaz Marije Krucifikse Kozulić 3, 51000 Rijeka, Croatia,
info@intechopen.com or visit our website at intechopen.com.

Meet the editors

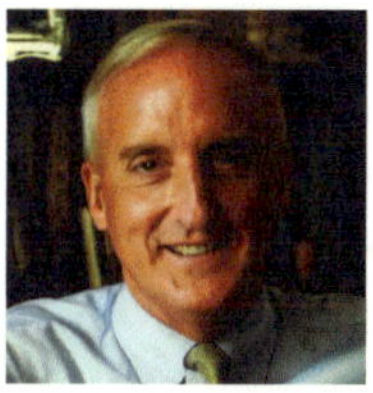

Peter Clark, SJ, Ph.D., is the John McShain Chair in Ethics and Director of the Institute of Clinical Bioethics at Saint Joseph's University, Philadelphia, USA. He is also the bioethicist for the Jefferson Health System, St. Christopher's Hospital for Children and Shriners Hospital for Children, Philadelphia, USA, Our Lady of Lourdes Hospital, Mercy Hospital, Baltimore, USA, Catholic Charites of Maryland, Community Suburban Hospital, and Caritas Baby Hospital, Bethlehem, Palestine. As a bioethicist, Dr. Clark is responsible for the ethical training of the medical fellows, residents, and interns in all the acute care hospitals. He does weekly ethics teaching rounds at the three acute care hospitals in the Jefferson Health System Northeast and Suburban Community Hospital; he co-chairs the hospital ethics committees, IRBs and the Corporate Ethics Committee and is on consult 24/7 for all the hospitals. Dr. Clark received his Ph.D. in Medical Ethics from Loyola University, Chicago, USA, and is the author of numerous articles in medical and bioethics journals on topics including medical futility, pain management, prejudice in the medical profession, the medical use of marijuana, safe injection sites, opioid prevention and education, tube feedings and PVS patients, male circumcision and HIV/AIDS, face transplantation, and the Ashley treatment, among others. He is also the author of *To Treat or Not to Treat: The Ethical Methodology of Richard A. McCormick as Applied to Treatment Decisions for Handicapped Newborns and Death with Dignity: Ethical and Practical Considerations for Caregivers of the Terminally Ill. Dr. Clark is also editor of Contemporary Issues in Bioethics and Bioethics: Medical, Ethical and Legal Perspectives*. Dr. Clark is also a reviewer for numerous bioethics journals and is a member of various medical and ethical organizations nationally and internationally.

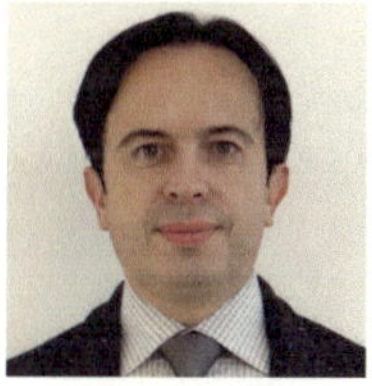

Kamil Hakan Dogan, MD, Ph.D., is a Full Professor and Chair in the Department of Forensic Medicine, Faculty of Medicine, Selcuk University, Turkey. Dr. Dogan received his MD from the Faculty of Medicine, Gazi University, Turkey, in 2000. After his extensive research in forensic medicine, he received his Ph.D. in Biochemistry in 2012. He gives lectures on forensic medicine and medical ethics to medical students as well as students of the dentistry and law faculties. He is the editor of five books and the *Bulletin of Legal Medicine* and a reviewer for several international journals. He has published more than 200 articles in refereed journals, chapters in textbooks, and abstracts in scientific meetings.

Contents

Preface

The field of bioethics is a relatively new discipline that is becoming more complex by the day. As science continues to advance, ethical questions are being exposed, and few in the scientific field seem interested in taking the time to discern whether we should do all that can be done. Just because something can now be accomplished, does that mean we should move forward and allow it to advance? Bioethicists are the ones raising the "red flags" about issues that are a concern to them and to society as a whole. These issues are complex, and the complexity involves areas of medicine, science, law, and ethics. Should we move forward with genetically modified pig kidneys in humans? Should we create children from three persons when the mitochondria from the biological mother are defective? Is medical rationing inevitable? Should we genetically modify children? When does personhood begin? Should therapeutic medical procedures be allowed to develop into enhancement procedures? When do medical treatments become medically futile? Has autonomy become absolute in medicine today? Are patients/proxies dictating medical treatments? Why are so many medical articles being retracted by journals? How safe are genetically modified foods? When is a new pharmaceutical discovery too expensive for society? Should we implant chips in the brain to improve people's ability to think and move? Should CRISPR be used to alter the genes of babies? Should we transfuse synthetic blood that would enhance performance by increasing speed, strength, and endurance? Can paediatricians discharge a minor from their practice because they refuse vaccinations? Should we implant computer chips in patients to track their locations? These questions and more are being debated by scientists, lawyers, politicians, and bioethicists around the world, but the fear is that the scientists will succeed in advancing these new procedures and technologies because biotechnology corporations see a profit to be made by implementing them.

There seems to be a real distrust of science and corporations in regard to science-related topics. Many fear the end results. Will the future involve a new dividing point: the enhanced versus the unenhanced? Who will be able to afford these new procedures? The fear is these new techniques will cause a greater divide in the world between the "haves" and the "have-nots". This divide already exists, and we cannot afford for the divide to widen.

The safety of these new procedures and techniques needs to be examined in depth. Long-term implications and consequences need to be considered because the future of humanity hangs in the balance. The long-term health effects of these procedures need to be scrutinized. The implications of how these new procedures will impact the quality of the environment must be considered. The public is beginning to realize that science is impacting various aspects of humanity, including climate change, childhood vaccinations, genetically modified foods and animals, responsible research with nonhuman primates, and more. The issue is that there must be a group of responsible individuals who are willing to be at the forefront of these scientific gains in order to question, challenge, and debate the scientists to make sure that the future of humanity is protected and will be treated with dignity and respect. It is the role of the bioethicist today to engage in a constructive dialogue with colleagues in medicine, scientific research, pharmaceutical and biotech firms, and law so that new procedures and techniques are completely vetted from all vantage points to preserve and defend the very dignity and respect of the human person. This job may appear daunting at first, but unless those trained in philosophical and theological ethics take the lead, the future of humanity will be compromised. This book is an attempt to encourage a dialogue with our colleagues in medicine, research, and law to examine these critical bioethical issues from all sides so that the best interests of patients, families, and society will be protected in the future.

Peter Clark, Ph.D.
John McShain Chair in Ethics,
Director-Institute of Clinical Bioethics,
Saint Joseph's University,
Philadelphia, Pennsylvania, USA

Kamil Hakan Dogan
University Faculty of Medicine,
Department of Forensic Medicine,
Selçuk University,
Konya, Turkey

Section 1

Legal Perspectives

Chapter 1

(Legal) Status of Embryo in Biomedically Assisted Procreation

Urban Vrtacnik

Abstract

Legal and ethical theories see different approaches to the status of the embryo (full status, no status, limited status). The latter conception is upgraded with proportionality status in which the level of rights increases with gestational development. The development of assisted reproduction techniques (ART) from the late 1970s onward led us to the uncharted territories. The status of the embryo (fetus) is no longer debated only in relation to spontaneous conception and development in the mother's womb but also in relation to the procedures in vitro. Therefore, issues related to embryo storage (surplus embryos), embryo research, and genetic diagnostics shall be examined in the course of the following chapter, along with different approaches to the protection of the (early) embryo in international and domestic laws. The final part shall be dedicated to the discussion on how to regulate the status of the embryo *de lege ferenda*, also acknowledging further developments in ART.

Keywords: medical law, bioethics, embryo, ART, IVF

1. Introduction

Modern medical law and bioethics has strongly evolved around issues of reproductive medicine since its very beginnings. It has to be noted in this respect that renowned Joseph Fletcher's Harvard lectures from the 1949 already included ethical issues on artificial insemination [1] after the first reports on the human artificial insemination came from Guttmacher—1943, Stoughton—1948, and Kohlberg—1953 [2]. Fletcher's lectures shall be considered as first academic inputs in contemporary (reproductive) ethics, while the term "bioethics" was not even commonly used until the late 1960s [1]. Another milestone came with the first baby born as a result of in vitro fertilization in 1978 (Steptoe and Edwards, UK), which was not seen only as a revolution in the medical sense but it also brought strong reflections in the fields of social studies. Creation of human life outside of the mother's womb, new family liaisons (in case of donor involvement), IVF related research and diagnostics, potential abuses in manipulation with human tissues and cells, and so on were the topics that gained importance in the course of the development of reproductive medicine. The pioneers of IVF, Steptoe and Edwards, noted already in 1980 that IVF procedures "*brought hope to thousands of* (infertile) *couples*," but at the same time, they triggered "*interests to millions* of *others watching from the sidelines*" [3]. I may add, in such respect (and more than 40 years later), that IVF (along with accompanying medical procedures) showed us not only how life can be conceived in a new manner (and thus prevent involuntary childlessness for many infertile couple) but also how to handle equilibrium between progress and security in every (biomedical) conduct, related with genetic material. In the late 1980s and early 1990s, legislative documents on biomedically assisted reproduction were adopted throughout Europe (e.g., Norway—1987, UK—1990, Germany —1991, Austria—1991, France—1994), whereas in 1997, we saw the signing of Oviedo convention (the Convention for the Protection of Human Rights and Dignity of the Human Being with regard to the Application of Biology and Medicine), which is the only international legally binding instrument on the protection of human rights in the biomedical field to date [4].

Since any procreation (spontaneous or biomedically assisted) is inseparable with the embryo being conceived, it comes with no surprise that (legal) status of the embryo is strongly debated in contemporary law and bioethics. It attracts several issues from prevention of pregnancy, termination of pregnancy, assisted reproductive techniques (ART), embryonic research, embryonic stem cells, and so on. Some of the authors even acknowledge the status of the embryo as one of the most important legal, ethical, and moral issues of the present time [5].

This chapter firstly provides definition of the embryo (fetus), in both medical and legal sense. Then, it gives insight into various positions (statuses) of the embryo, from the full status and limited status to the no (zero) status. When it comes to the proportionality status (observed within the limited status), this chapter also briefly reveals the stages of embryotic (fetal) development and discusses the connection between the phases and potential level of rights acquired. Finally, it touches the questions of dignity of the embryo, mostly in relation to "surplus" embryos, embryo research, and embryonic diagnostics.

This chapter stays within the boundaries of medical law and ethics, while further discussion is needed within the legal profession as well as in interaction with other sciences and social studies.

2. Definition of the embryo and legal theories

Medical science recognizes the human embryo in every development of human fertilization from the stage of the mitosis (zygotic splitting) onward. In the theory of embryogenesis, the first stage (zygote) appears approximately 8 hours after the fertilization (fusion of sperm cells and ovum). As the diploid cell, the zygote includes separate genetic material of the parents, whereas the transcription of DNA happens in the next stage (mitosis) to form two-cell structure (embryo in biological sense). This is followed by 4- and 8-cell cleavage and finally morula (16–32 cell cleavage). The morula is further developed into blastocyst, which is consistent of outer cell mass (trophoblast), blastocyst cavity (blastocoele), and inner cell mass (embryoblast). From the latter, embryo is further developed [6, 7].

Legal definition of the embryo follows the medical doctrine (the crucial point of existence of embryo is regularly set to the point of time when it acquires its unique DNA); however, it makes some exceptions when considering assisted reproduction. Whereas the nidation of the embryo into the mother's womb is possible at the stage of blastocyst by spontaneous conception, embryo transfers in IVF treatments can be done earlier, from the two-cell structure onward [7]. Therefore, legal protection of the embryo may come earlier in relation to ART, even in the zygotic phase. This was significant for the first UK HFE Act from 1990 [8], which differentiated embryo (every stage of human development from fertilization) from live embryo, which matched the stage of executed fertilization at the stage of the zygote. Amendments to HFE Act (HFE Act 2008), however, settled the definition that *"embryo means a live human embryo"* and *"references to an embryo include an egg* (oocyte) *that is in the process of fertilization or is undergoing any other process capable of resulting in an embryo"* [9]. Similarly, Slovenian legislation—Infertility Treatment and Procedures of Medically Assisted Reproduction Act from 2000—ZZNPOB [10] stipulates that embryo is conceived when oocyte is fully fertilized, while "early embryo" includes zygote and embryo that develop outside of the mother's womb no longer than 14 days or until the primitive streak is formed. It is commonly understood, in such respect, that the zygote has to acquire and retain potential for further embryonic development to enjoy legal protection [4]. In any moment in which such development comes to an end, legal protection in the sense of the special regime under reproductive legislation ceases, respectively. Contrary to that, German reproductive legislation, and bylaws, as well as guidelines of the Medical Chamber, which importantly influenced regulatory landscape in Germany [4], recognize the embryo no earlier than in stage of mitosis but allows the manipulation and storage of zygotes in ART to avoid prohibition on maximum number of embryos being transferred into the mother's body (see below). Oviedo convention does not provide direct definition on the embryo but forbids the use of techniques of medically assisted procreation for the purpose of choosing a future child's sex (except where serious hereditary sex-related disease is to be avoided) and the creation of human embryos for research purposes. It also stipulates that, where the law allows research on embryos, it shall ensure adequate protection of the embryo [11]. Predominant early legal protection of the embryo in ART is also in line with a contemporary biological definition that considers that human embryo is a discrete entity, which has arisen from either *(i) the first mitotic division when fertilization of a human oocyte is complete or (ii) any other process that initiates organized development of a biological entity with a human nuclear genome or altered human genome that has potential to develop up to, or beyond, the stage at which the primitive streak appears* [12]. This is in line with predominant legal definitions of the embryo (in European countries), which are based on the idea of "potentiality"—cell or group of cells to be capable of generating a human being [13]. When considering the legal status of embryo, European Court of Justice (ECJ) also provided its own definition. It was adopted when ECJ deliberated on the patentability of embryo pluripotent stem cells according to the EU Directive 98/44/CE in Oliver Brüstle v Greenpeace eV. case. According to ECJ, the embryo is *any human ovum after fertilization, any non-fertilized human ovum into which the cell nucleus from a mature human cell has been transplanted and any non-fertilized human ovum whose division and further development have been stimulated by parthenogenesis* [14]. All these definitions offer solid grounds to assess "embryo rights" in every legal position, especially considering statuses that will be described below. Additionally, it may be observed that every definition makes a reference to the further embryonic development, meaning that embryo in ART has to have potential to further develop (in vitro) and finally (in vivo), leading to birth deriving from biomedically assisted conception. This is recognized as both the ultimate therapeutic goal and a legal good of interest.

After being aware of the embryo definitions, it has to be further assessed whether the embryo enjoys the status of the human being, and further, does it accrue (acquire) legal personality—capacity to have rights and obligations? It has to be noted in such respect that "personality" in the legal sense means entitlement to rights and obligations, whereas "a person" in a common sense is seen as individual with its intellectual, emotional, and spiritual qualities, which are manifested in relation to others.

Similarly, a "human being" in the biologically sense is a member of human race (conceived through fertilization of human gametes), whereas broader (also theological) views encompass physical (body) and spiritual (soul) elements of the human being. Furthermore, "rights" in the legal sense used in this chapter represent the persons' ability to act or be defended (protected) in a certain way defined by the law, whereas actions or protective measures can be commissive or omissive [4]. As already mentioned in the introduction, theory recognizes different legal statuses of the embryo, which follow basic moral statuses as introduced in contemporary bioethics [15]. *Full status* means that the embryo enjoys exact same level of rights as the born person; *no (zero) status* means that the embryo enjoys no rights (and it is therefore considered merely as an object), whereas the *limited status* is resting somewhere between full and zero status. This means that the embryo can acquire certain rights but not all the rights of a born person. The most popular limited position is the *proportional status* position, which holds that the level of rights increases with gestational development until full scope of rights are acquired at birth and beyond [15]. If legislative solutions (and commonly adopted principles and rules of bioethics) are observed, we see that full status is not prevailing in predominant part of the jurisdictions worldwide [4, 16–18]. Since the right to life is seen as absolute and non-waiver right (often reflected in the constitutional term of inviolability of human life), full recognition of the full status would impose that every (medical, surgical) abortion, certain manners of contraception (used in the past [5, 19]), as well as certain procedures in ART (especially when "surplus" embryos are discarded after not being transferred to the woman's uterus) would be recognized as a violation of the right to life and consequentially classified as a murder [4]. It also becomes critical that the embryo cannot express its genuine will (capacity or ability to choose between different possible courses of action unimpeded); therefore, full status would make every embryonic research and diagnosis practically impossible, since medical measures and research on humans strictly require informed consent of the person (subject) to which the procedure refers (whereas potential limited capacity of the embryo already departs from the full status in question). In the European legal theory (and also theory of bioethics), it is therefore recognized that the embryo does not enjoy full (constitutional) rights, especially not those related to inviolability of the human life [16–18] and potentially also not those related to protection (inviolability) of physical and mental integrity. Therefore, full status can be seen more of an ideal (considering the moral position of sanctity or uniqueness of life), to which we shall strive in the specific case or specific position (topos), while it cannot be accepted as the general approach. It has to be noted somehow that absence of recognition to the full status does not mean that legal restrictions shall not apply in relation to the embryo. There are some restrictions that aim to protect the position of embryo to the maximum extent possible, usually just until the collision with constitutional rights of the others (e.g., freedom of choice in childbearing, healthcare rights, horizontal dignity). However, this situation already falls within the limited status, as it will be highlighted below.

Furthermore, there are not many authors who would uphold zero status either. Žnidaršič made a great statement when saying that it seems irrational that a fully developed embryo would hold absolutely no rights 1 day prior to birth, while 1 day later it would acquire all the rights [5]. It becomes evident in such respect that the lapse of the very short time prior the birth is not in any way (legally) significant in the course of embryonic development. Therefore, it is seen contrary to the general ethics and common morals (and also contrary to the law, if I may add) that we would freely dispose with such fully developed embryo just prior to the birth. I add to this position, however, that the embryo, irrespective of the phase of embryonic development, holds a unique genetic code (since the mitosis onwards) and therefore the potential to be developed into a (individual and unique) human being. This certainly calls at least for the limited status to be observed, which is also a concept widely used in legal theory and in many jurisdictions [4, 15].

Constitutional status that is most common associated with the position of the embryo (within the limited status) is dignity. Since the dignity is generally seen as a recognition of the value of humanity (human life, human potential) as such, it certainly matches the position (status) of the embryo as described above. Legal theoretics in the field of Constitutional law say that "*dignity affirms the same natural endowment of everyone with all that humans value.* In this context, "everyone" is seen as the "*heir of the past rational action of all members of society and a potential participant in all future positive achievements of humanity*" [20]. Certain constitutional systems therefore openly recognize constitutional right of embryo to dignity (including Slovenian [4]), so do the international documents, namely, Protocol I to the Oviedo Convention on the Prohibition of Cloning Human Beings [21]. The said Protocol clearly aims to protect the dignity and identity of all human beings, including embryos. Therefore, it may be dignity that could be at utmost importance in the light of the most relevant topics in contemporary assisted reproduction (surplus embryos, embryo diagnostics, embryo research, see the next section). While the dignity is predominantly seen as the right of the specific person, it triggers correlative duty (of the state, other individuals) to protect such dignity, namely, to value human potential to the maximum extent possible. In the light of the cotemporary bioethics, such approach to dignity is seen more as *dignity as empowerment (rights-based dignity that vests dignity in autonomous choice constrained only by the rights of the others)* rather than as *dignity as constraint* (*which considers dignity to the extent beyond autonomous choice and permits constraint on individuals to protect their interests or the interests of the community*) [15]. Those two concepts, however, may not be fully or directly transferable to the debates on embryo since the embryo lacks common ability to make autonomous choice. This makes evaluation on the legal status even more difficult, considering the fact that individuals, who are not able to express their will, usually require more (legal) protection or higher level of awarded rights than the others. And further, dignity as empowerment also has its inevitable limitations, since the right of autonomous choice (of minors and adults) also derives from the human dignity itself, which inevitably leads us to the horizontal collision on human rights. The dignity within the limited status shall not be confused with certain views associated with "dignitary alliance" which go in favor of (absolute) sanctity and inviolability of life (which is mostly associated with the full status position) but is closer with more widely accepted dignitarism, which *inter alia* promotes the principle that human life should not be commodified (e.g., with sex selection, reproductive cloning, savior siblings), nor commercialized (precluding the sale of human bodies or body parts, commercial surrogate motherhood, patenting of normal gene sequences, etc.) [see 22].

At the end of this section, certain thoughts need to be dedicated also to the proportionality status. For the purposes of this chapter, we used the term embryo for the whole course of the gestational development from the conception until birth. However, it cannot be overlooked that medical science recognizes the transfer from the embryonal to the fetal phase at approximately **eight (8) weeks** into the pregnancy. Therefore, we shall use term "fetus" from the 8 weeks of the pregnancy onward if we strive to be terminologically correct. It should be also noted that until the end of the **week 8** of the pregnancy, the head of the baby is already formed, neural tube along the back is closed, there are certain buds that are to become limbs, and fingers have begun to form. Furthermore, during the **(i) week 9–12**, we can observe development of muscles, nerve system, respiratory system, heartbeat, brainwaves, first development of eyes, members; **(ii) after week 18**, fetus might begin to hear; **(iii) after week 23**, the fetus gains possibility of living outside of the mother's body, responding to voices; **(iv) after week 24**, we can see formation of lungs; and **(v) after week 28**, there comes capability of autonomous breathing, while **(vi) after week 37**, we consider fetus as mature [23]. Therefore, questions of (allowed) interference into physical and physiological integrity of fetus (along with the protection of its dignity) come into the equation under the proportionality status. This also matches the reason why many jurisdictions impose gestational limit for (non-indicated) abortion on request, which is usually set between **10** and **14 weeks** [24, 25]. Proportionality is therefore a status that is already applicable in certain (protective, limitative) measures, which go in favor of the embryo (even if legal capacity of the latter is acquired no earlier than at the birth). However, such debate clearly exceeds the scope of this chapter. Procedures of biomedically assisted reproduction namely end with the transfer of the embryo into the woman's uterus (also referred to as "objective time limits of biomedical assistance in conception" [4]), while after such transfer, the general (no longer special) rules of embryo protection shall apply. Similarly, general obstetrics would be the medical area that would replace reproductive medicine once the pregnancy is achieved. Since there is no significant change in the gestational development from the conception (mitosis) to the embryo transfer (being related to any differences in legal status of the embryo or the level of its rights), we believe there is no further need to explore the status of proportionality in relation to ART.

3. Surplus embryos, embryo research, embryo diagnostics

The first area in biomedically assisted reproduction, where the question of dignity of the embryo will be raised as essential, is the area of creation of embryos outside the mother's body, their storage, and their further use. In such context, we encounter the question of the so-called *surplus embryos*, which is seen as one of the focal issues in reproductive medicine. With IVF procedures, a larger number of embryos can be formed outside the mother's body (due to the larger number of removed gametes with the aim of maximizing the success of the IVF procedure), whereas due to various legal restrictions (e.g., the number of embryos that can be transferred into the woman's body or the total the number of IVF cycles available), it may happen that certain embryos (which may even be biomedically suitable and therefore have potential to result in pregnancy) are not being transferred into the woman's body. Such embryos are called "surplus" or "spare" embryos [15], whereas the disposal of such embryos undoubtedly constitutes interference with the right to dignity. As already explained above, the embryo holds the genotypic characteristics of the future human being and therefore embodies potential to be developed in a person with individual physical, personal, and spiritual qualities. The path to the possible future person may be therefore ended (and the human value inevitably lost) with each disposal of the surplus embryo.

European regulations tackle those issues differently. In some countries, the number of embryos that are allowed to be created outside the body in one cycle shall match the exact number of transferred embryos into the woman's body (e. g., in Germany, meaning no more than three embryos can be cryopreserved, since maximum of three embryos are allowed to be transferred per cycle, [4]), while in some other countries, the number of oocytes that can be retrieved in a single cycle is limited (to three oocytes, Croatia, [4]), which automatically limits the maximum number of the embryos created and potentially cryopreserved (no more than three per cycle). In some countries, it is not possible to start a new IVF cycle until all the embryos that are stored have been transferred into the woman's body (France, [4]), whereas in some other countries, repeated embryo transfers are possible within the same (reimbursable) IVF cycle if the pregnancy is not achieved within previous attempts (Slovenia, [4]). In those countries, there is no absolute (numeric) limitation on the number of embryos that are allowed to be cryopreserved [4]. In some countries, the possibility of donating embryos was also made available under certain statutory conditions (Great Britain, France, Croatia, Netherlands [4, 26]), which of course goes in favor of respecting the human value and human potential of the embryo. However, each of the solutions also brings some disadvantages. Solutions by limiting the number of embryos may result in the reduced efficiency of IVF procedures and therefore in narrowing of reproductive rights, which fall within the protection of the family life—right to found a family [27]. It has been namely confirmed by the clinical studies in the past that repetition of IVF cycles has positive impact on cumulative delivery rates, almost leveling the delivery potential of the general population with the population of certain groups of infertile couples [4, 28]. Similarly, limiting the possibility of embryo storage may also bring some drawbacks, since it may result in undesired practical solutions that are not consistent with the intention of the legislator. Such situation was seen in the German case when freezing of zygotes (which was not directly prohibited by the law) was chosen instead of embryo storage (see above and [4]), meaning that the problem was solved only provisionally, since disposal of "surplus zygotes," under the condition that they are or may be developed into embryos, makes no less interference into the dignity as in the case of surplus embryos. This may also call for the early protection of the embryo (or protection of the "early embryo"), as described above. Solutions related to embryo donation, on the other hand, depend entirely on the decision and willingness of the partners to donate embryos, while they also raise certain ethical concerns in the direction of the benefit of the child, who in the case of embryo donation has no biological connection with any of his genetic parents [4]. The Dutch report also mentioned (even though it clearly highlighted satisfactory effect to the embryo recipients) that delivery rates in embryo donation showed limited success (12.6%), partly due to high pregnancy loss through miscarriage and partly due to inferior freezing techniques [26]. Mentioned solutions do not entirely solve the problem of surplus embryos; however, they help to considerably limit either the number of embryos conceived and/or the number of the embryos disposed. It can be also empirically observed that combination of different legislative measures may be beneficial since it may be more successful in leveling advantages and drawback within accrued benefits. Another missing puzzle in the subject matter lies in the fact that the majority of jurisdictions does not include reference to the protection of dignity of embryo in the legislative documents; however, this has not prevented legislative solutions to evolve and ameliorate to date in the sense of the better embryo protection. This also refers to reimbursement policies, which still vary in European countries [4]. We do believe that fully reimbursable IVF cycles (sufficiently repeated, along with covered costs of cryopreservation) may not only prevent discrimination on the grounds of economic status (in relation to the prospect to found a family) but also have positive effect on the issue of surplus embryos.

Another major area related to the issue of the dignity of embryos is the issue of research involving embryos and embryo diagnostics. In relation to *research on (early) embryos*, it should be noted that national legislations in Europe predominantly contain relatively strict provisions, which are the result of the awareness that the issues of research work on germ cells and embryos are sensitive, and it is therefore necessary to avoid inadmissible instrumentalization and commercialization in relation to genetic material [4]. On the international regulatory side, the first (and so far, the only) binding regulation relating to the human rights in biomedicine is Oviedo Convention. The intention of the convention was to provide direct (binding) effects in the jurisdictions of the signatory countries; however, in several places, the convention explicitly refers to regulation by national law. The nature of the Convention is therefore directly binding (for the signatory countries in which Convention acts as a regulation), but at the same time, there are a number of areas that are left to further instrumentalization in national legislation. Concerning the regulation on human genome, Oviedo convention includes provisions on nondiscrimination on the grounds of genetic heritage (Article 11), conditions for predictive genetic tests (Article 12, see also below), limitations on interventions on the human genome (Article 13), and prohibition on the selection of sex (Article 14). On the other hand, thc provisions related to *research on embryos in vitro* (Article 18 of) are relatively scarce. Oviedo convention namely stipulates only that: (i) the creation of human embryos (author's note: *only*) for research purposes is prohibited, and (ii) where the law allows research on embryos in vitro, it shall ensure adequate protection of the embryo. Such scarce provisions (without even specifying the standard of "adequate protection") are a consequence of large (irreconcilable) disagreements between individual countries, members of the Council of Europe when adoption Oviedo convention [4]. Therefore, the question on whether an individual country will allow research on embryos or not and under what conditions is predominantly left to national legislative arrangements. It has to be added, however, that regardless of this supranational position, every embryo research in the national context, if permitted by the law, should also be compliant with Article 15, 16, and 17 to Oviedo convention, which provides general conditions on any scientific research in the field of biology and medicine. In such context, *research on a person* (mutatis mutandis the embryo) may only be undertaken: (i) if there is no alternative of comparable effectiveness to research on humans; (ii) if the risks which may be incurred by that person are not disproportionate to the potential benefits of the research; (iii) if the research has been approved by the competent body after independent examination of its scientific merit, including assessment of the importance of the aim of the research and multidisciplinary review of its ethical acceptability (usually done by national research ethics committee - NREC); and (iv) if persons undergoing research have been informed of their rights and the safeguards prescribed by law, and the informed consent was given (expressly, specifically, and being documented). Such consent may be freely withdrawn at any time. Conditions under Oviedo Convention have to be met cumulatively [11]. When speaking of the embryo (and its inherent rights), it is debatable on how the embryo can provide informed consent, since it is not capable to express its own will in any way. The answer to such question shall be found within the national laws. Speaking of the Slovenian legal system, the written informed consent of the couple (man and woman who undertake procedures of biomedically assisted reproduction) is sufficient. It has to be added that embryo research in Slovenia is only allowed for the purposes of protection or improvement of the human health (medical purpose) and only when research procedures cannot be efficiently executed in animal embryos or alternatively

(Article 38 to Slovenian Infertility Treatment and Procedures of Medically Assisted Reproduction Act—ZZNPOB [10]). In addition to approval of the NREC, special permit of the National commission for biomedically assisted reproduction is needed. Additionally, the research is permitted only on embryos, which are not suitable for the transfer into the mother's body or storage, as well on surplus embryos that would be discarded under statutory conditions (Article 38 of ZZNPOB). It is evident that conditions for embryo research vary from country to country (pursuant to the framework of Article 18 to Oviedo Convention); however, Slovenian legislation gives a clear example that national may include rather strict provisions on embryo research, which may even exceed the level of (overall) protection provided (guaranteed) by Oviedo Convention.

Finally, part of the discussion should also be devoted to issues related to embryo diagnostics, especially PGT(−M) and PGT-A procedures (previously also known as PGD and PGS procedures). Preimplantation genetic testing for monogenic/single gene disease—PGT(−M) includes procedures for the targeted identification of known severe hereditary or genetic disease that the embryo could have due to the health condition or genetic characteristics of the parents. On the other hand, preimplantation genetic testing for aneuploidy—PGT-A is an examination to determine any genetic defect or disease of the embryo, regardless of the indication that would arise from the medical history of the parents [4, 29]. Both types of genetic diagnostics are inextricably linked to assisted reproduction (the procedure can be performed in vitro, most often by the ICSI method), whereas such procedures may (also) be performed on couples who would otherwise be capable to conceive a child spontaneously. Genetic diagnostics therefore constitute a method of assisted reproduction, which is not (necessarily) medically indicated on the basis of infertility but is based on the medical goal to prevent the transmission of a severe hereditary disease to the child. In this context, the duty of the state, with the right associated with the procedures assisted reproduction, is understood not only in the direction of ensuring the possibility of infertile couples to realize their parenthood (the right to found a family) but also in preventing the birth of children who could have serious hereditary diseases.

Supranational regulatory grounds for genetic testing of the embryo can be found in Article 13 to Oviedo convention, which stipulates: *Tests which are predictive of genetic diseases or which serve either to identify the subject as a carrier of a gene responsible for a disease or to detect a genetic predisposition or susceptibility to a disease may be performed only for health purposes or for scientific research linked to health purposes, and subject to appropriate genetic counseling*. This means that the Oviedo convention allows genetic diagnostics under the provided conditions, whereas other terms are (again) left to be regulated within national legislation. Additionally, derivative details on the conditions applicable may also vary from country to country (as per type of disease, severity of disease, required consequences on the health of child, etc.), which may impose several differences in access to genetic testing through Europe [4]. However, it is commonly accepted that PGT-M (previously PGD) procedures are compliant with the right to dignity of the embryo and its position in the framework of the human rights. PGT-M (through biopsy of the embryo) can namely only take place on the basis of a medical indication on the part of the parents and with the legitimate goal of preventing the birth of a child with a serious genetic disease. At the same time (if the transfer of genetic disease is ruled out through PGT-M), the life potential of the embryo is safeguarded. Contrary to that, PGT-A procedures are not allowed in certain European countries (e.g., in France, Germany, Norway, Slovenia), as their performance does not require proof of a real, above-statistical risk for the existence of a serious illness, being potentially transferred to the child (therefore, such PGT-A procedure is considered as a blind test). This may indirectly lead to the process of selecting of embryos without a prior medical indication, which may be contrary to the provisions of the Oviedo convention. "Genetic counseling" in a sense of Article 13 of the Oviedo Convention is namely understood as giving information on how genetic conditions might affect you or your family, which is done on a basis of personal or family (medical) history. Also, such PGT-A procedures (together with the associated procedures of assisted reproduction) are ethically questionable, mostly for the lack of the medical utility. Both partners (especially the woman) may be namely exposed to the assisted reproduction procedures (which interfere in physical and mental integrity), without the existing (proven) medical reason for doing so. There are some serious risks to a woman's health in ART, with both stimulation of the ovaries and oocytes retrieval (hyperstimulation, damage to neighboring organs), which seem to not outweigh the goal deriving from nonproven risk of a disease being transferred to the child. This, of course, does not refer to infertile couples, which undertake IVF in any way (due to their infertility). Therefore, in the context of the discussion regarding the ethical principle of (medical) utility, we may see the PGT-A procedures (with no genetic counseling) as contrary to the basic principles of medical ethics.

However, some further ethical and legal dilemmas may be also raised in relation to PGT-M procedures. If we make a short detour into the literature, the poem of Aldous Huxley's entitled Fifth Philosopher's Song' from 1920 reads:

A million million spermatozoa.

All of them alive;

Out of their cataclysm but one poor Noah.

Dare hope to survive.

And among that billion minus one.

Might have chanced to be.

Shakespeare, another Newton, a new Donne—.

But the One was Me.

Shame to have ousted your betters thus,

Taking ark while the others remained outside!

Better for all of us, froward Homunculus,

If you'd quietly died! [30].

Huxley gives a great reference to the uniqueness of every human life, even before birth, linking such uniqueness with living potential (*Might have chanced to be)* and mere individuality (the uppercase letter in *"Me"* is intentionally used in such context). If such "Me" is negated, since it is discarded as a consequence of PGT-M (confirming the possibility of the transmission of a severe genetic disease from the parents to the child), the individual human value is inevitably and irreversibly lost. The slippery slope argument even increases, if we consider that some authors report that the probability of a *wrong diagnosis* in PGT-M is up to 5% [31], while some other authors report that such probability is even up to 10% [15]. This means that, in a certain percentage, the described diagnosis can prevent the realization of life potential and nullifies the uniqueness of future life of a completely healthy embryo (person). This means that due to a *statistical* error, the one "who could have been Me" will never be born. On the other hand, we should not overlook that the main goal of PGT-M is to protect the dignity and health of the future child, which is endangered if the child is born with a serious illness. This is based on a belief that dignity (as a value of the human being) is negatively affected in case of severe illnesses (related to unbearable suffering), which can be avoided in advance by medical measures (diagnostics). Among serious illnesses (which may be transferred from parents to the children), the theory often mentioned conditions associated with an extremely poor quality of life or/and early mortality (e.g., in cystic fibrosis, Lesch–Nyhan syndrome, hemophilia, and Duchenne's muscular atrophy). The probability of such diseases in a child can undoubtedly be predicted with PGT-M. Given that the regulation in assisted reproduction strictly aims to health protection and care for the benefits and rights of (future) children [4], the same (necessarily) relates to PGT-M, also considering provisions of Oviedo Convention. In addition to that, European Court of Human Rights already stipulated (in Costa and Pavan v. Italy case) that even the parents (in the context of the right to privacy and family life according to Article 8 of the ECHR) enjoy an independent right to conceive a child who does not have serious health problems [32]. Since such right may be not dependable on the economic status of the parents (to avoid unjust discrimination on the said grounds), we believe that such right can be properly effectuated only in environments that guarantee full reimbursement of IVF procedures required to perform genetic diagnostics (PGT-M). It can be thus concluded that in the context of ethical and constitutional weighing, the benefits of (fully reimbursable) PGT-M outweigh the risks and weaknesses of such procedures. Based on that, the existing regulations of genetic testing of the embryo (including the conditions set in favor of the protection of the embryo and the protection of the health and welfare of the future child) can be observed as appropriate. However, in the future, the increase in the reliability of PGT-M will certainly contribute to the fact that the ethical risks arising from such diagnostics will decrease.

4. Conclusion: way ahead in embryo status (and protection)

This chapter showed us that the definitions of embryo are well settled in medical as well as in legal practice. Certain significance is associated with procedures of assisted reproduction, where the protection of the embryo may come earlier, from the zygotic phase onward, under condition of further embryonic development. Such approach also had impact on the contemporary general medical definition as well as on the case-law related to the legal definition of the embryo. Yet again, the environment of assisted reproduction showed the way to the general approaches in medicine, law, and ethics. Furthermore, the scope of rights of the embryo is predominantly settled within the limited status, whereas dignity, physical and mental integrity, as well as the health protection are the rights to be observed in such respect. The proportionality status does not have a large impact on assisted reproduction; however, it becomes crucial in general limitations and safeguards related to any (medical, research) conducts related to the embryo. Issues on surplus embryos, embryo diagnostic, and research are deliberated on supranational and national levels. Speaking of the latter, national legislations include rather strict regulation on embryonic research, whereas in the field of genetic diagnostics, PGT-M procedures are predominantly observed as legitimate and ethically accepted.

Lastly, it should be emphasized that the issue of the status of the embryo is a distinctly interdisciplinary issue, which means that in terms of competence, it will be a matter of division between the fields of philosophy, theology, (bio)medicine, embryology, and law. Solely legal and medical or embryological science will not be able to independently offer definitive answers to the questions asked in the future. This shall become crucial in the development of assisted reproduction where the new procedures (e.g., uterus transplantation, artificial uterus) and new manners of embryo diagnostics (e.g., in prevention of infectious diseases, assessing a future child as a potential donor) will certainly open new ethical and legal debates. Rather than *constitutio translativa*, in the sense of shifting the burden of finding solutions to other sciences or social studies, it will be *constitutio definitiva*, since all the aforementioned sciences will have to find a consensus regarding the proposed (legal) solutions. These will not only be, of course, seen as a reflection of professional findings but also depend on social and political conditions.

Author details

Urban Vrtacnik[1,2]

1 Law Firm Vrtacnik, Ljubljana, Slovenia

2 Faculty of Law, University of Maribor, Maribor, Slovenia

*Address all correspondence to: urban@vrtacnik.si

References

[1] Jonsen AR. A Short History of Medical Ethics. Oxford, New York: Oxford University Press, Inc.; 2008

[2] Ombelet W, van Robays J. Artificial insemination history: hurdles and milestones. Facts, Views & Vision ObGny. 2015;7(2):137-143

[3] Edwards R, Steptoe P. A Matter of Life. London: Hutchinson & Co. (Publishers) Ltd; 1980

[4] Vrtacnik U. Legal Aspects of Biomedical Assistance in Procreation [Thesis]. Univerza v Ljubljani: Pravna fakulteta v Ljubljani; 2018

[5] Žnidaršič Skubic V. Civilno medicinsko pravo: izbrane teme. Ljubljana: Uradni list Republike Slovenije; 2018

[6] Petrovič D. Normalen razvoj človeškega zarodka in nepravilnosti v njegovem razvoju. Medicinski razgledi. 2003;**24**:184

[7] Virant Klun I, Tomaževič T. Od nastanka gamet do rojstva: oploditev z biomedicinsko pomočjo: teoretični in slikovni prikaz nastanka gamet, zgradbe gamet in tehnik oploditve z biomedicinsko pomočjo. Radovljica: Didakta; 2002

[8] United Kingdom of Great Britain and Northern Ireland. Human Fertilisation and Embryology Act 1990 [Internet]. Available from: https://www.legislation.gov.uk/

[9] United Kingdom of Great Britain and Northern Ireland. Human Fertilisation and Embryology Act 2008 [Internet]. Available from: https://www.legislation.gov.uk/

[10] Republic of Slovenia. Infertility Treatment and Procedures of Medically Assisted Reproduction Act – ZZNPOB. Official Gazette of the Republic of Slovenia, No. 70/2000 w/amendments

[11] Council of Europe. The Convention for the Protection of Human Rights and Dignity of the Human Being with regard to the Application of Biology and Medicine: Convention on Human Rights and Biomedicine (Oviedo Convention). Council of Europe, 1998; Official Gazette of the Republic of Slovenia, No. MP 17/98 w/amendments

[12] Findlay JK, Gear ML, Ilingworth PJ, Junk SM, Kay G, Mackerras AH, et al. Human embryo: A biological definition. Hum Rep. 2007;**22**:905-911. DOI: 10.1093/humrep/del467

[13] De Miguel BI. What is a human embryo? Croatian Medical Journal. 2014;**55**:669-671. DOI: 10.3325/cmj 2014.55.669

[14] European Court of Justice (ECJ). Judgment of the Court (Grand Chamber) of 18 October 2011; Oliver Brüstle v Greenpeace eV.: Case C-34/10. European Court Reports 2011 I-09821

[15] Pattinson SD. Medical Law and Ethics. 4th ed. London: Sweet & Maxwell - Thomson Reuters; 2014

[16] Beauchamp TL, Childress JF. Principles of Biomedical Ethics. 5th ed. New York: Oxford University Press; 2001

[17] Stauch M, Wheat K, Tingle J, editors. Text, Cases and Materials in Medical Law and Ethics. 4th ed. New York: Routlege; 2012

[18] Zupančič K. Oploditev z biomedicinsko pomočjo: O osnutku naših predpisov. In: Polajnar Pavčnik A,

Wedam Lukić D, editors. Medicina in pravo. Ljubljana, Cankarjeva Založba; 1998. pp. 237-244

[19] Wicks E, editor. Human Rights and Healthcare. Oxford: Hart Publishing; 2007

[20] Šturm L, editor. Komentar Ustave RS. Ljubljana, FPDEŠ Ljubljana; 2002

[21] Council of Europe. Additional Protocol to the Convention for the Protection of Human Rights and Dignity of the Human Being with regard to the Application of Biology and Medicine, on the Prohibition of Cloning Human Beings. Council of Europe, 1998; Official Gazette of the Republic of Slovenia, No. MP 17/98 w/amendments

[22] Trontelj J. Spoštovanje človekovega dostojanstva v zvezi z biomedicino: mednarodni dokumenti in slovenski pravni red. Bogoslovni vestnik. 2004;**64**(3):517-529

[23] Mayo Clinic, Pregnancy by week [Internet] 2023. Available from: https://www.mayoclinic.org

[24] Centre for reproductive rights. European Abortion Laws: A Comparative Overview [Internet]. Available from: https://reproductiverights.org/

[25] De Zordo S, Zanini G, Mishtal J, Garnsey C, Ziegler AK, Gerdts C. Gestational age limits for abortion and cross-border reproductive care in Europe: a mixed-methods study. BJOG: An International Journal of Obstetrics and Gynaecology. 2021;**128**(5):838-845. DOI: 10.1111/1471-0528.16534

[26] Pieters JJPM, van Miltenburg MHAM. Altruistic Donation of Surplus Embryos to Known and Unknown Recipients, The Dutch Approach. Int. International Journal of Fertility and Sterility. 2022;**16**(3):230-236. DOI: 10.22074/IJFS.2022.538120.1183

[27] Council of Europe. Convention for the Protection of Human Rights and Fundamental Freedoms (European Convention on Human Rights), Council of Europe, 1950; Official Gazette of the Republic of Slovenia, No. MP 7-41/1994 w/amendments

[28] Vrtacnik U, Bokal Vrtacnik E, Devjak R. Cumulative Delivery Rate after Providing Full Reimbursement In Vitro Fertilization Programme: A 6-Years Survey. BioMed Research International. 2014;**2014**:850478. DOI: 10.1155/2014/850478

[29] Sciorio R, Tramontano L, Catt J. Preimplantation genetic diagnosis (PGD) and genetic testing for aneuploidy (PGT-A): status and future challenges. Gynecological Endocrinology. 2020;**36**(1):6-11

[30] Huxley A. Fifth Philosopher's Song. 1920. [Internet] Available from: https://www.oxfordreference.com

[31] Joksimovič Č. Predimplantacijska genetska diagnostika. Bolnišnica za ženske bolezni in porodništvo Postojna. Postojna; 2002. [Internet] Available from: https://docplayer.gr

[32] European Court of Human Rights (ECHR). Costa and Pavan vs. Italy: Judgement No. 5470/10 of August 28th, 2012 [Internet]. Available from: https://www.hudoc.echr.coe.int

Chapter 2

Balancing Equity and Autonomy: The Utilitarian Case for the Public Funding of Non-Invasive Prenatal Testing in Hong Kong

Wai-King Tsui, Yuk-Chiu Yip and Ka-Huen Yip

Abstract

Non-invasive prenatal testing (NIPT) demonstrates superior performance compared to conventional screening methods currently available within Hong Kong's public healthcare system. Nevertheless, the substantial costs associated with NIPT render it inaccessible for much of the population, leading to ethical debates surrounding public funding. A conflict emerges between the imperative to allocate limited resources efficiently and the obligation to uphold ethical principles of equity and reproductive autonomy within the public healthcare system. Adopting a utilitarian-based approach, this chapter initially presents three central arguments suggesting that NIPT can be ethically integrated into the public healthcare system. Subsequently, the discussion examines the challenges associated with incorporating NIPT into Hong Kong's strained public healthcare system. To address these challenges, we propose two potential solutions: (1) introducing NIPT as a second-tier screening test for high-risk pregnancies, or (2) offering NIPT through public-private partnerships, which would alleviate the demand on public sector resources. Implementing a nominal fee for NIPT adheres to the principle of impartiality in public resource allocation, ensuring equitable decision making without favoring specific population groups. Ultimately, the future of NIPT in Hong Kong necessitates expanding its availability, enhancing its accuracy, and incorporating it into comprehensive prenatal care. This approach will support the reproductive autonomy of pregnant women and promote accessible healthcare.

Keywords: non-invasive prenatal testing, prenatal screening, healthcare ethics, women's health, public healthcare

1. Introduction

1.1 Non-invasive prenatal testing: background, clinical application, and accessibility in Hong Kong

Non-invasive prenatal testing (NIPT) is a screening test that involves analyzing the fetal genome using cell-free fetal DNA (cfDNA) samples from maternal blood.

The term "non-invasive" refers to the method of obtaining the cfDNA sample; during pregnancy, the fetus releases some of its DNA into the maternal bloodstream, which can be analyzed through testing a blood sample obtained from the mother to assess for the presence of chromosomal abnormalities and determine the baby's risk for a number of genetic disorders [1]. The relative frequencies of Down's syndrome (Trisomy 21), Edwards' syndrome (Trisomy 18), and Patau's syndrome (Trisomy 13) in the general population are 1 in 500, 2.3 in 10,000, and 1.4 in 10,000, respectively [2].

Before the invasive confirmatory diagnostic tests, the Hospital Authority of Hong Kong currently provides two prenatal screening tests specific to the trimester of pregnancy as first-tier screening tests for assessing the risk of Down's syndrome. These tests involve ultrasound scans and blood tests and are offered during the first and second trimesters of pregnancy. The first-trimester screening test is conducted at 11–13 weeks and detects approximately 80–90% of Down's syndrome pregnancies. The second trimester screening is conducted for pregnancies between 14 and 20 weeks and detects around 80% of Down's syndrome pregnancies. However, when compared with NIPT, these two prenatal screening tests are less accurate and more time-consuming. NIPT offers several advantages over the conventional screening tests [3]. It is more accurate and reliable, with relatively low false-positive rates [1]. Additionally, NIPT is much safer than invasive prenatal diagnosis tests or chorionic villus sampling (CVS), which are usually performed at later gestational periods in the second trimester (12–20 weeks). NIPT can be performed as early as 10 weeks of pregnancy, and the results can be obtained within 5–7 days.

Currently, NIPT is not offered by the Hospital Authority of Hong Kong but can be accessed through the Chinese University of Hong Kong Fetal Medicine Private Clinic and other private clinics. This screening test is most often provided on a self-financed basis as prenatal screening, costing around 5000 HKD in private clinics. Private practitioners and commercial laboratories provide most of these services [4]. However, due to the high cost of the test, few women or couples can afford it. The public funding of NIPT could enable all women and couples to have equal access to NIPT and ensure that their reproductive autonomy is not limited by their financial status.

1.2 Aims of this chapter

Given the Hospital Authority's ongoing efforts to introduce NIPT into public maternal services, this chapter aims to conduct a utilitarian-based analysis of the ethical issues relevant to the local context of Hong Kong, to examine compelling arguments for the matter. Specifically, in a prior discourse [5], we highlighted the necessity for a theory-driven framework to facilitate the ethical implementation of NIPT as a screening modality. This chapter builds upon our previous discussion and extends the scope of the conversation to encompass the pragmatic aspects of enacting utilitarian-based arguments within a public healthcare system.

2. Overview of public and private prenatal care in Hong Kong

The healthcare system of Hong Kong is a dual-track system comprising private and public sectors, overseen by the Department of Health and the Hospital Authority respectively. Primary care is largely provided by private doctors, who offer more prompt service but at increased cost. In contrast, the public sector furnishes comprehensive care and serves as the main provider of secondary and tertiary healthcare, including outpatient clinics and general hospitals. Expectant mothers accessing the private system can choose and consistently consult with the same physician and hospital, albeit at significantly higher fees. Under the current system, women may utilize a combination of both sectors, obtaining prenatal examinations and supplemental ultrasounds from the public system while also visiting a preferred private doctor.

In the public sector, the Obstetrics and Gynecology Departments of hospitals under the Hospital Authority collaborate with the Maternal and Child Health Centers (MCHCs) of the Department of Health to provide affordable antenatal shared-care to expectant mothers, costing just a few hundred dollars. This includes health education, maternal and fetal health checkups, tests and ultrasounds, labor, birth care, and aftercare for mothers and babies. Expectant mothers receive specialist care from healthcare professionals and attend regular antenatal checkups at a nearby MCHC. Antenatal care also includes routine screening tests for Universal Down's Syndrome and Group B Streptococcus, with additional tests conducted for expectant mothers with abnormal results or special clinical needs. In the public sector, midwives attend most of the births. Although public maternity care is less expensive, the wait at government maternal clinics can be long and appointments are often brief.

3. Ethical issues and competing values related to NIPT

The ethical issues related to NIPT result from the question of whether the introduction of NIPT to the public healthcare system conforms to ethical values, which sometimes compete with one another. These ethical values are crucial to the assessment of medical ethics:

3.1 Choice, autonomy, and informed consent

A foundational ethical principle in medicine is respecting patient autonomy through informed consent. This means patients should make voluntary decisions regarding medical tests and procedures based on comprehensive, unbiased facts presented in clear, understandable language. Consent cannot be considered fully informed if patients do not adequately comprehend the information furnished to them.

With innovative prenatal genetic tests like NIPT, clinicians have an obligation to take extra care in educating expectant mothers on how the procedure works, what conditions it screens for, its benefits and limitations, and possible test results. This empowers women to make autonomous, informed choices about their pregnancy care. However, achieving truly informed consent for NIPT poses challenges. Complex genetic terms must be explained in plain language that patients can understand. The conditions screened for should be clearly described so patients fully comprehend what is being tested. Patients must also understand that NIPT is a screening tool, not a diagnostic test, and have its limitations clearly explained. Additionally, they need to grasp the possible results and options available following different outcomes.

To overcome these challenges, clinicians are advised to take time to explain NIPT and associated concepts in straightforward, easy-to-understand language at approximately a 5th grade reading level. The goal is to present information on NIPT in a way that facilitates patient comprehension while still maintaining medical accuracy. Using language appropriate for a 5th grade reading level allows the use of common, everyday words while avoiding patronizing oversimplification. Going lower than 5th grade risks distorting key details and sacrificing important nuances. For clinicians' consideration, specific techniques to improve patient understanding include breaking down complex terms and explaining genetic concepts simply, using graphics or illustrations to demonstrate how NIPT works, and having patients explain their understanding of what NIPT is, how it works, its purpose, benefits, and limitations. Any gaps or inaccuracies in patient explanations can be clarified by reviewing the information again. This process may be repeated, depending on patients' level of understanding. Clinicians may ask patients to teach back certain key facts about NIPT to demonstrate reasonable comprehension prior to making an informed decision about consenting to the test.

3.2 Avoidance of harm (non-maleficence)

It is the responsibility of the government to minimize or eradicate any harm caused by healthcare interventions, whether they are provided in public or private sectors. This duty involves ensuring that healthcare providers adhere to safety guidelines and take necessary steps to prevent harm to patients.

3.3 Equality, inclusion, and fairness (justice)

The government is obligated to uphold equality and fairness by implementing policies that combat prejudice, bias, and discrimination. A crucial aspect of fulfilling this duty is ensuring that public funds are fully utilized for these purposes.

The advent of non-invasive prenatal testing (NIPT) has raised several ethical concerns regarding the tension between enhancing individual reproductive autonomy and protecting the interests of society as a whole. On one hand, NIPT promotes pregnant women's reproductive autonomy by furnishing them with information to make informed choices about their pregnancies. However, this autonomy relies on access to unbiased details about the test and the conditions screened. Furthermore, some ethicists worry that NIPT could infringe on the future autonomy of fetuses as individuals. NIPT may also reduce harm by replacing more invasive procedures, but inaccurate results could negate this benefit by causing undue anxiety and prompting further testing. Moreover, a significant reduction in the incidence of genetic conditions due to NIPT could diminish research funding and services for affected groups, potentially marginalizing them. Conversely, by empowering informed reproductive choices, NIPT could promote equality. However, funding NIPT publicly could conflict with fair resource allocation. Additionally, NIPT may set narrower boundaries on what constitutes a healthy pregnancy, stigmatizing disabled individuals and families. Overall, realizing the benefits of NIPT while mitigating ethical pitfalls will require nuanced policymaking that balances individual rights and ethical values.

4. Integrating NIPT into the public healthcare system: a utilitarian lens

Utilitarianism is an ethical theory that evaluates actions based on their consequences. As originally formulated by Jeremy Bentham in the eighteenth century, utilitarianism aims to maximize overall happiness by quantifying the utility of each action's positive and negative effects on the people involved [6]. John Stuart Mill later refined utilitarianism in the nineteenth century by emphasizing the qualitative aspects of happiness and considering the social utility of actions, not just individual utility [7]. There are two main branches of utilitarianism: act utilitarianism judges individual acts based on their utility, while rule utilitarianism focuses on adhering to moral rules that tend to produce the greatest utility overall [8, 9].

When considering public funding for non-invasive prenatal testing (NIPT), utilitarianism provides a useful framework for weighing the potential benefits and harms. Widespread access to NIPT through public funding could maximize utility by empowering pregnant women to make informed reproductive choices and detect fetal abnormalities early in pregnancy. However, the unlimited use of NIPT may negatively impact societal welfare if applied unethically, such as for sex selection of fetuses based on certain cultural preferences. Therefore, a utilitarian approach would support implementing rules and limitations on NIPT usage to ensure it promotes the greater good. The principle of beneficence, emphasizing the well-being of pregnant women, should be central when formulating healthcare policies on NIPT provision. With appropriate safeguards in place, offering NIPT through a public healthcare system can be ethically justified under utilitarianism by maximizing its advantages for the population while minimizing the risks of misuse.

For the ethical use of NIPT in public healthcare, three arguments have been established.

4.1 Argument 1: pregnant women who opt for NIPT after informed decision-making should be provided with the test since it is a reliable and valid prenatal screening tool. NIPT offers essential information that empowers women to make autonomous decisions regarding their reproductive health

Argument 1 is based on the fact that NIPT offers pregnant women reliable and accurate information about fetal aneuploidy in the early stages of pregnancy. A recent meta-analysis of high-quality data has shown that NIPT has a high degree of accuracy in detecting trisomy 13, 18, and 21 across various obstetrical populations [10]. Additionally, a negative result [11] from NIPT is highly dependable and provides reliable information about fetal aneuploidy as early as the 10th week of pregnancy. Furthermore, results from NIPT are typically available within 7 days [12]. Therefore, NIPT empowers pregnant women to make informed reproductive choices by facilitating the decision-making process [13–15]. Indeed, NIPT allows pregnant women more time to consider other prenatal tests or reproductive interventions, as a positive result from NIPT is informative enough to make decisions even without follow-up confirmatory testing. This longer period for decision-making allows for thoughtful consideration of available options, earlier monitoring of fetal development, consulting relevant professionals to address any concerns related to a positive result, and the chance to plan and make arrangements for the delivery and care of a child with a disability.

Argument 1 asserts that undergoing NIPT should be a matter of informed choice, as pregnant women have the right to decline information about fetal aneuploidy, even if present. An informed choice is a decision based on relevant knowledge, consistent with the decision maker's values, which is behaviorally implemented [15, 16] and crucial for enhancing reproductive autonomy [17–19]. Being informed allows pregnant women to make a choice that respects their right not to know, as they should be made aware that the results of the NIPT may lead them to face unexpected choices, which they might want to avoid [20]. A pregnant woman should understand the scope, limits, purpose, potential risks, and implications of NIPT [21]. The absence of an informed decision regarding NIPT can compromise reproductive choices and autonomy for women [20].

4.2 Argument 2: NIPT should be delivered based on its favorable utility profile, and non-directive genetic counseling should be provided before and after the testing process

Undergoing NIPT for prenatal screening of fetal aneuploidy has the potential to bring a variety of benefits to pregnant women, as well as some risks [20, 22]. These benefits include reduced maternal anxiety over fetal health if the test yields a negative result [17], a lower need for invasive follow-up tests with their associated 0.1–0.2% risk of miscarriage [17, 23], and a reduced likelihood of unanticipated births of children with aneuploidy [24]. NIPT also enables less physically risky and less emotionally traumatic decisions regarding the termination of pregnancy at an earlier stage [25], and it can be performed without an upper limit for gestational age, allowing women who present late for their first prenatal visit to take the test without resorting to other screening modalities with lower sensitivity and specificity rates [26]. Undergoing NIPT is associated with significantly less fear of pain and discomfort compared to amniocentesis or CVS [27], and it could be offered in more settings compared to invasive methods; indeed, a maternal blood sample can be obtained by a nurse while obtaining samples for CVS and amniocentesis require the specialized skills of a physician [28, 29]. Furthermore, it allows women to prepare for an affected child, and it may be used as a preliminary test to help women in deciding if they wish to engage in further invasive tests [30].

However, potential risks may also be present, such as unreliable test results leading to misguided optimism [19, 24]. While reproductive geneticists consider false-negative results from NIPT to be uncommon, false-positive outcomes (with a probability of around 0.1%) can occur due to factors like placental mosaicism, obesity in the person being tested, presence of a maternal tumor, or ethnicity, particularly if the person is of Afro-Caribbean descent. Additional concerns may also arise from incidental findings that lack clear clinical significance. Despite these risks, ethicists generally agree that NIPT displays a superior and advantageous utility profile as a prenatal screening test [17]. Serious professional organizations including the American College of Obstetrician and Gynecologists, the International Society for Prenatal Diagnosis, and the National Society of Genetic Counselors endorse the implementation of NIPT in prenatal screening within healthcare systems. They suggest that the advantages and usefulness of NIPT outweigh the associated risks for pregnant women [31].

The normative claim for Argument 2 is that, from a utilitarian perspective, the offer of a prenatal screening test is ethically justified if it maximizes utility with minimal associated risks. In other words, the morally right action is the one that produces the most favorable balance of good over evil. The utilitarian view for NIPT in prenatal screening is that offering NIPT within the public healthcare system is ethical depending on how we can maximize the benefits of NIPT while minimizing the associated risks. The ethical framework of the United Nations Educational, Scientific, and Cultural Organization aligns with this utilitarian perspective and stipulates that for a prenatal testing offer to be ethically acceptable, the benefits or utility, in this case, must outweigh the drawbacks [18].

Along with the compelling and advantageous utility profile of NIPT, non-directive genetic counseling before and after the testing is also recommended. This would help to maximize positive outcomes and reduce unwanted risks, aligning with the utilitarian's perspective on the ethical implications of offering NIPT in a public healthcare system. Several studies have demonstrated that pre-test and post-test counseling by trained professionals can help pregnant women exercise autonomy in making reproductive decisions regarding the acceptance of a positive or negative NIPT result [19, 22, 32–34].

4.3 Argument 3: utilitarianism favors the offer of NIPT with a small fee, and for the less financially capable group of pregnant women, government subsidies should be provided to maximize the number of beneficiaries

According to this argument, offering free-of-charge NIPT may not necessarily provide the highest utility for pregnant women. Requiring a nominal fee from test recipients is more appropriate as it discourages ill-considered testing, which could undermine the usefulness of the test. Some literature has expressed concern about the adverse ethical consequences of ill-considered testing, especially with regards to the primary objective of NIPT to promote reproductive autonomy [20]. Research suggests that asking women to pay for prenatal screening enhances their awareness related to the need to make an informed choice before undergoing the test [35].

Government subsidies for NIPT for less financially capable pregnant women may broaden the scope of beneficiaries within the public healthcare system. Some studies have theorized that reproductive health is a collective responsibility, and that governments have a role to play in promoting reproductive health at a population-wide level [17, 36]. Utilitarianism should support the provision of government subsidies to enable economically disadvantaged groups to undergo NIPT, facilitating access to NIPT for the largest possible number of women who could potentially benefit from the test.

Beyond the advantageous utility profile of NIPT, utilitarianism requires that the maximum number of pregnant women should derive benefits from the test. While some may argue that the proposed small fee for NIPT may lead to the marginalization of less financially capable women, this underscores the idea that maximum utility can only be achieved through unrestricted availability of the test, with the local government (i.e., taxpayers) assuming the societal cost of providing fundamental prenatal care. Offering free-of-charge NIPT may result in hasty decisions, impeding the desired effect of promoting reproductive autonomy. Therefore, utilitarians would agree that providing government subsidies to financially disadvantaged women may be necessary to expand to a larger base of beneficiaries who can access the test while providing a safety net for those who need it.

5. Enabling choices and reproductive autonomy amid healthcare system's finite resources

As indicated by prior research [20], non-invasive prenatal testing (NIPT) serves not as a means to reduce the birth of children with Down's syndrome, but rather as a tool to support women's autonomy in reproductive decision making. NIPT carries broader societal implications beyond merely evaluating the risks and benefits for expectant mothers. However, within the context of Hong Kong's constrained public healthcare system due to limited human resources, exclusively offering NIPT through public healthcare services without alternative measures would compromise autonomy and choice. Given the inadequate pre-test and post-test counseling resources for pregnant women, they may feel compelled to make certain decisions based solely on test outcomes, rather than exercising free choice regarding reproductive autonomy. In terms of cost effectiveness, providing NIPT to all expectant mothers within a strained public healthcare system is not a fiscally prudent decision. One potential solution for maximizing NIPT's social utility in light of healthcare resource challenges is the establishment of public-private partnerships.

Hong Kong's public health services, particularly secondary and tertiary care, are increasingly transitioning aspects of service delivery to private sector involvement. Notable examples include the 2008 Cataract Surgery Program, a public-private partnership in which participating patients receive approximately 5000 HKD subsidy for cataract surgery performed by private ophthalmologists, and the 2010 Hemodialysis Public-Private Partnership Program, which enables eligible patients with end-stage renal disease to access financially subsidized services from private hemodialysis providers. Similarly, the operational philosophy and model of these programs could be applied to NIPT, allowing pregnant women to choose between subsidized private sector care or public sector care. This strategy not only grants pregnant women greater autonomy of choice but also alleviates the burden on the public healthcare system and optimizes NIPT's social utility.

When incorporating NIPT into Hong Kong's existing public healthcare system, it is prudent to consider the limitations of resources, particularly human resources. Additionally, providing adequate pre-test and post- test counseling may be challenging due to the myriad possible outcomes associated with false-positive Down's syndrome screening results. If NIPT were to replace current prenatal screening tests as first-tier screening tests, a sudden surge in demand for the highly sought-after genetic counseling service would likely ensue. Without access to well-informed, accurate, and balanced information about NIPT, satisfying the first two established arguments would prove difficult. This concern can be addressed by introducing NIPT as a second-tier screening test for women whose first-tier ultrasound scans and blood tests indicate a risk of congenital abnormalities in their unborn child. Alternatively, when employing NIPT as a first-tier screening test, it could be offered through public-private partnerships akin to the Cataract Surgery Program. This approach would substantially reduce public sector demand for NIPT, allowing existing public resources to meet the demand.

Regarding the third argument, it is unlikely that requiring pregnant women to pay a nominal fee for the favorable utility profile would encounter significant public objection, as the number of affected women would be relatively small. Moreover, imposing a fee would support the principle of impartiality in public resource allocation, ensuring fair and just decision-making that balances the interests of various population groups without demonstrating partiality or preference towards specific individuals. The future trajectory for NIPT in Hong Kong may involve expanding its availability, enhancing its accuracy, and integrating it more fully into routine prenatal care. This development has the potential to contribute to more comprehensive and accessible prenatal care for pregnant women in Hong Kong.

6. Conclusion

To maximize the social utility of NIPT as a prenatal screening modality within Hong Kong's public healthcare system, it is crucial to address ethical considerations, public funding, and resource allocation. Utilitarianism presents three arguments that can guide public policymakers in ensuring the optimization of NIPT's social utility over time.

DOI: http://dx.doi.org/10.5772/intechopen.1002945

Introducing NIPT into Hong Kong's public healthcare system poses challenges due to limited resources, particularly human resources. Providing adequate pre-test and post-test counseling could be challenging (for example, due to the multitude of possibilities associated with false-positive Down's syndrome screening results). If NIPT were to replace current prenatal screening tests as first-tier screening tests, a sudden surge in demand for the highly sought-after genetic counseling service would occur. Without access to well-informed, accurate, and balanced information about NIPT, satisfying the first two established arguments becomes difficult. This concern can be addressed by introducing NIPT as a second-tier screening test for women whose first-tier ultrasound scans and blood tests indicate a risk of congenital abnormalities in their unborn child. Alternatively, when employing NIPT as a first-tier screening test, it could be offered through public-private partnerships, greatly reducing the demand for NIPT in the public sector and allowing current public resources to cope with the demand. Regarding the third argument, it is unlikely that requiring pregnant women to pay a nominal fee for the favorable utility profile would encounter significant public objection, as the number of affected women would be relatively small. Moreover, imposing a fee would support the principle of impartiality in public resource allocation, ensuring fair and just decision-making that balances the interests of various population groups without demonstrating partiality or compassion towards specific individuals.

In conclusion, providing NIPT to all expectant mothers in Hong Kong through public healthcare services may not represent the most viable solution due to limited resources. However, public-private partnerships offer a pragmatic alternative that addresses the challenges posed by the strained public healthcare system and supports women's reproductive autonomy. By following the examples of the Cataract Surgery Program and the Hemodialysis Public-Private Partnership Program, NIPT can be made more accessible, integrated into routine prenatal care, and alleviate public healthcare resource burdens. This strategy grants pregnant women greater autonomy of choice and ensures that NIPT's social utility is maximized. Ultimately, the future of NIPT in Hong Kong lies in expanding its availability, enhancing its accuracy, and integrating it into comprehensive prenatal care, thus supporting the reproductive autonomy of pregnant women and fostering more accessible healthcare.

Funding

None.

Conflict of interest

The authors declare no conflict of interest.

Notes/thanks/other declarations

None.

Author details

Wai-King Tsui[1], Yuk-Chiu Yip[2] and Ka-Huen Yip[1*]

1 Caritas Institute of Higher Education, Hong Kong, China

2 Hong Kong Metropolitan University, Hong Kong, China

*Address all correspondence to: khyip@cihe.edu.hk

References

[1] Mazloom AR, Džakula Ž, Oeth P, Wang H, Jensen T, Tynan J, et al. Noninvasive prenatal detection of sex chromosomal aneuploidies by sequencing circulating cell-free DNA from maternal plasma. Prenatal Diagnosis. 2013;**33**:591-597. DOI: 10.1002/pd.4127

[2] Savva GM, Walker K, Morris JK. The maternal age-specific live birth prevalence of trisomies 13 and 18 compared to trisomy 21 (Down syndrome). Prenatal Diagnosis: Published in Affiliation with the International Society for Prenatal Diagnosis. 2010;**30**(1):57-64. DOI: 10.1002/pd.2403

[3] Yi H, Hallowell N, Griffiths S, Yeung LT. Motivations for undertaking DNA sequencing-based non-invasive prenatal testing for fetal aneuploidy: A qualitative study with early adopter patients in Hong Kong. PLoS One. 2013;**8**(11):e81794. DOI: 10.1371/journal.pone.0081794

[4] Benitez MA. Hong Kong's public hospitals to offer non-invasive Down's syndrome test for free to women with high-risk pregnancies [Internet]. South China Morning Post. 2018. Available from: https://www.scmp.com/news/hong-kong/health-environment/article/2143753/hong-kongs-public-hospitals-offer-non-invasive [Accessed: January 22, 2023]

[5] Yip YC, Tsui WK. Ethical considerations for offering non-invasive prenatal tests within a public healthcare system: A rule utilitarian perspective. Ethics & Medicine. 2020;**36**(2):101-167

[6] Driver J. The history of utilitarianism. Stanford Encyclopedia of Philosophy. 2009. Available from: https://plato.stanford.edu/entries/utilitarianism-history/

[7] Cahn SM, editor. Seven Masterpieces of Philosophy. New York: Routledge; 2016. DOI: 10.4324/9781315508818

[8] Horty JF. Perspectival act utilitarianism. In: Dynamic Formal Epistemology. Dordrecht: Springer Netherlands; 2010. pp. 197-221. DOI: 10.1007/978-94-007-0074-1_11

[9] Eggleston B, Miller DE, Weinstein D. John Stuart Mill and the Art of Life. Oxford: Oxford University Press; 2011. DOI: 10.1093/acprof:oso/9780195381245.001.0001

[10] Gil MM, Accurti V, Santacruz B, Plana MN, Nicolaides KH. Analysis of cell-free DNA in maternal blood in screening for fetal aneuploidies: Updated meta-analysis. Ultrasound in Obstetrics & Gynecology. 2017;**50**:302-314. DOI: 10.1002/uog.17484

[11] Greene MF, Mello MM, Morain S. A new era in noninvasive prenatal testing. The New England Journal of Medicine. 2013;**369**(22):2165. DOI: 10.1056/NEJMp1304843

[12] Boon EM, Faas BH. Benefits and limitations of whole genome versus targeted approaches for noninvasive prenatal testing for fetal aneuploidies. Prenatal Diagnosis. 2013;**33**(6):563-568. DOI: 10.1002/pd.4111

[13] de Jong A, de Wert GM. Prenatal screening: An ethical agenda for the near future. Bioethics. 2015;**29**(1):46-55. DOI: 10.1111/bioe.12122

[14] Lau JY, Yi H, Ahmed S. Decision-making for non-invasive prenatal testing

for down syndrome: Hong Kong Chinese women's preferences for individual vs relational autonomy. Clinical Genetics. 2016;**89**(5):550-556. DOI: 10.1111/cge.12743

[15] Lewis C, Hill M, Chitty LS. Women's experiences and preferences for service delivery of non-invasive prenatal testing for aneuploidy in a public health setting: A mixed methods study. PLoS One. 2016;**11**(4):e0153147. DOI: 10.1371/journal.pone.0153147

[16] Marteau TM, Dormandy E, Michie S. A measure of informed choice. Health Expectations. 2001;**4**(2):99-108. DOI: 10.1046/j.1369-6513.2001.00140.x

[17] Dondorp W, de Wert G, Bombard Y, Bianchi DW, Bergmann C, Borry P, et al. Non-invasive prenatal testing for aneuploidy and beyond: Challenges of responsible innovation in prenatal screening. Summary and recommendations. European Journal of Human Genetics. 2015;**23**(11):1438-1450. DOI: 10.1038/ejhg.2015.56

[18] International Bioethics Committee of the United Nations Educational, Scientific and Cultural Organization. Report of IBC on updating its reflection on the human genome and human rights [Internet]. 2015. Available from: https://unesdoc.unesco.org/ark:/48223/pf0000233258 [Accessed: January 22, 2023]

[19] Wertz DC, Fletcher JC, Berg K. Review of ethical issues in medical ethics [Internet]. World Health Organization. 2003. Available from: https://apps.who.int/iris/handle/10665/68512 [Accessed: January 22, 2023]

[20] Kater-Kuipers AB, Bunnik EM, De Beaufort ID, Galjaard RJ. Limits to the scope of non-invasive prenatal testing (NIPT): An analysis of the international ethical framework for prenatal screening and an interview study with Dutch professionals. BMC Pregnancy and Childbirth. 2018;**18**(1):1-4. DOI: 10.1186/s12884-018-2050-4

[21] Biesecker BB, Schwartz MD, Marteau TM. Enhancing informed choice to undergo health screening: A systematic review. American Journal of Health Behavior. 2013;**37**(3):351-359. DOI: 10.5993/ajhb.37.3.8

[22] Vanstone M, King C, de Vrijer B, Nisker J. Non-invasive prenatal testing: Ethics and policy considerations. Journal of Obstetrics and Gynaecology Canada. 2014;**36**(6):515-526. DOI: 10.1016/S1701-2163(15)30568-5

[23] Oepkes D, Page-Christiaens GC, Bax CJ, Bekker MN, Bilardo CM, Boon EM, et al. Trial by Dutch laboratories for evaluation of non-invasive prenatal testing. Part I—Clinical impact. Prenatal Diagnosis. 2016;**36**(12):1083-1090. DOI: 10.1002/pd.4945

[24] Bianchi DW, Wilkins-Haug L. Integration of noninvasive DNA testing for aneuploidy into prenatal care: What has happened since the rubber met the road? Clinical Chemistry. 2014;**60**(1):78-87. DOI: 10.1373/clinchem.2013.202663

[25] Mentula MJ, Niinimäki M, Suhonen S, Hemminki E, Gissler M, Heikinheimo O. Immediate adverse events after second trimester medical termination of pregnancy: Results of a nationwide registry study. Human Reproduction. 2011;**26**(4):927-932. DOI: 10.1093/humrep/der016

[26] Chitty LS, Hill M, White H, Wright D, Morris S. Noninvasive prenatal testing for aneuploidy–ready for prime time? American Journal of Obstetrics & Gynecology. 2012;**206**(4):269-275. DOI: 10.1016/j.ajog.2012.02.021

[27] Locock L, Field K, McPherson A, Boyd PA. Women's accounts of the physical sensation of chorionic villus sampling and amniocentesis: Expectations and experience. Midwifery. 2010;**26**(1):64-75. DOI: 10.1016/j.midw.2008.02.002

[28] Nizard J. Amniocentesis: Technique and education. Current Opinion in Obstetrics and Gynecology. 2010;**22**(2):152-154. DOI: 10.1097/GCO.0b013e32833723a0

[29] Jenkins TM, Sciscione AC, Wapner RJ, Sarto GE. Training in chorionic villus sampling: Limited experience for US fellows. American Journal of Obstetrics and Gynecology. 2004;**191**(4):1288-1290. DOI: 10.1016/j.ajog.2004.03.038

[30] Langlois S, Brock JA, Wilson RD. Genetics Committee: Current status in non-invasive prenatal detection of down syndrome, trisomy 18, and trisomy 13 using cell-free DNA in maternal plasma. Journal of Obstetrics and Gynaecology Canada. 2013;**35**(2):177-181. DOI: 10.1016/s1701-2163(15)31025-2

[31] Dey M, Sharma S, Aggarwal S. Prenatal screening methods for aneuploidies. North American Journal of Medical Sciences. 2013;**5**:182-190. DOI: 10.4103/1947-2714.109180

[32] Hodgson J, Spriggs M. A practical account of autonomy: Why genetic counseling is especially well suited to the facilitation of informed autonomous decision making. Journal of Genetic Counseling. 2005;**14**(2):89-97. DOI: 10.1007/s10897-005-4067-x

[33] Seavilleklein V. Challenging the rhetoric of choice in prenatal screening. Bioethics. 2009;**23**(1):68-77. DOI: 10.1111/j.1467-8519.2008.00674.x

[34] Schwartz B, Schwartz B. The Paradox of Choice: Why More Is Less. New York: ECCO; 2004. Available from: https://www.researchgate.net/profile/Cledwyn-Fernandez/publication/321964178_The_Paradox_of_Choice_Why_More_Is_Less/links/5d034b2292851c874c650ae9/The-Paradox-of-Choice-Why-More-Is-Less.pdf

[35] Munthe C. A new ethical landscape of prenatal testing: Individualizing choice to serve autonomy and promote public health: A radical proposal. Bioethics. 2015;**29**(1):36-45. DOI: 10.1111/bioe.12126

[36] Health Council of the Netherlands. Screening: Between Hope and Hype [Internet]. 2008. Available from: https://www.healthcouncil.nl/documents/advisory-reports/2008/04/01/screening-between-hope-and-hype [Accessed: January 22, 2023]

Chapter 3

Revisiting the United States Abortion Law and the Legal Implications

Richmond Ekhosuehi Idaeho

Abstract

Generally, female reproductive rights include the right to reproduce, maternity protection and childcare, access to adequate health care facilities, including information, counseling, and services in the family. More specifically, the right to reproduction refers to a woman's right to decide whether or not to have children, whether to carry or terminate an unintended pregnancy, and to choose the family planning and contraception technique that she prefers. This article examines the exercise of this right in the light of recent development in the United States jurisprudence. It also reviews the legal implications of this development on women's reproductive rights and other social cum medical issues particularly in relation to human rights and the "right" of the unborn.

Keywords: women, reproduction, health, right, abortion, unborn, human, life, privacy, ethics, jurisprudence, policy, law, fetus, conception, embryo, viability

1. Introduction

The controversy on when a fetus (or foetus) becomes a living being has been recently resurrected in the United States of America (the "US" or "United States") justice administration and amongst the public both within and outside the United States. Prior to the decision of the US Supreme Court in the case of *Dobbs v. Jackson Women's Health Organization,*[1] the well settled law which was established in *Roe v. Wade*[2] and applicable to all the States in the US ("States"), was that a pregnant woman has a right to determine what happens to her pregnancy whether to keep it or abort it.

In order words, women were granted the reproductive freedom and legal right to abort any unwanted pregnancies. This age long right recently came under scrutiny when the US Supreme Court took a new position, *albeit* overturning the principle in *Roe v. Wade* which upheld the legal right to abortion. Why did the Court reverse

[1] No. 19-1392; 597 U.S., argued on 1st December 2021 and decided on 24th June 2022.

[2] 410 U.S. 113 (1973), where the US Supreme Court held that the Constitution of the United States guarantees a woman's right to have an abortion. See also *Planned Parenthood v. Casey*, 505 U.S. 833 (1992), which held that foetal viability, i.e., ability to survive outside the womb, begins within 24 weeks, before which time a woman had a choice to abortion as guaranteed by the rights to privacy under the Fourteenth Amendment to the US Constitution.

its decision in *Roe v. Wade*? To answer this question, it is imperative to examine first how *Roe*'s case became a defining factor in establishing the right to abortion in the American society.

2. Women's reproductive right in the United States: the right to abortion

Abortion was already legal in several States of the United States prior to the Supreme Court decisions in *Roe v. Wade*[3] and *Doe v. Bolton*[4] which decriminalized abortion nationwide in 1973. The rulings created a federally mandated and consistent framework for States' legislations on the issue of abortion. Additionally, they set a minimum window of time during which an abortion would be permitted, with varying levels of limitations through the course of the pregnancy. This fundamental structure, updated in *Planned Parenthood v. Casey*,[5] was officially maintained throughout the States in the United States, although actual accessibility to abortion clinics varied greatly from State to State due to the absence of abortion providers in many counties. The permissibility and decriminalization of abortion has made many rethink the sanctity of life in an attempt to resolve the debate on when a fetus can become human.

The question several people, including biologists, ethicists, and jurists, have tried to answer over time has been "when does life begin?" In order words, at what time of conception can a fetus be classified as a human being; or put differently at what time can a fetus be worthy of ethical and legal consideration. Before delving into the arguments, it is important to consider the concepts of "human being", the "human person" and "human rights" or otherwise "rights." In this regard, a "human being" or the "human person" is used in this context interchangeably to refer to a living thing with the features of a human or person, that is a *homo sapiens*. The concept of a "person" may be more complex to define than that of a "human", as the former is largely a philosophical term while the latter is a scientific term. Whereas a "person" is used to refer to a being with certain capacities and attributes, which includes life, soul, and consciousness, that is a sentient being. A "human" on the other hand, is used to describe a being which is part of the *homo sapiens* with certain features including life, soul, conscious thoughts, erect posture, complex brain, amongst others. For all intent and purposes and without going into the various philosophical and scientific theories and analysis of these concepts, a human being and a human person are one and the same.[6]

Rights as used in this context refers to human rights. That is the rights available to a human being. These rights are regarded as human rights because they enure to a person on the grounds of being human. The United Nations (UN) defines human rights as the "rights inherent to all human beings, regardless of race, sex, nationality, ethnicity, language, religion, or any other status. Human rights include the right to life and liberty, freedom from slavery and torture, freedom of opinion and expression, the right to work and education, and many more" [1]. These rights are available to all humans, irrespective of gender.

Thus, critical to this discourse is the right to life and liberty, on which the issues relating to the right of the unborn child and women's reproductive right lie. Although "people agree that women have the right to make reproductive decisions involving

---

[3] *Supra*.

[4] 410 U.S. 179 (1973).

[5] *Supra*.

[6] http://www.differencebetween.info/difference-between-person-and-human, accessed on 23 June 2023.

their own bodies, many debate if those decisions directly affect other humans' bodies. This dispute on when a human's life begins likely plays a role in Americans' ethical and legal positions on abortion" ([2], p. 2). In his attempt at answering *albeit* understanding the question, the author of the article "Biologists' Consensus on 'When Life Begins'" has approached the issue from the standpoint of biologists' conception of human life, which majority agreed that 'life begins at fertilization.' He then went ahead to scrutinize the issue using the David Hume's *is—ought* problem.

> *"'When does a human's life begin?' is subject to David Hume's classic is-ought problem since the question has two primary interpretations: the descriptive view (i.e., when is a fetus classified as a human) and the normative view (i.e., when ought a fetus be recognized as a person worthy of ethical and legal consideration). The is-ought fallacy is present in some pro-life stances that confuse the former for the latter such that a certain descriptive view necessitates a corresponding normative view (e.g., 'since a human's life begins at fertilization, fetuses are worthy of legal protection throughout pregnancy'). This fallacy is also present in some pro-choice stances that confuse the latter for the former such that a certain normative view necessitates a corresponding descriptive view (e.g., 'since fetuses are not worthy of legal protection, a human's life begins at birth'). Careful consideration of the specific language used in a stance on when life begins is required to understand which interpretation drove that stance....*
>
> *This is-ought analysis can explain why people disagree on when life begins. Disagreement might not emanate from different biological views on when to classify a fetus as a human or different judgments on when a fetus is deserving of legal consideration. Conflicting stances could merely represent that one person interprets 'when life begins' descriptively while the other interprets it normatively. Thus, Americans could merely disagree because they understand the question differently." ([2], pp. 2–3)*

Hence, the arguments on 'when life begins' contributes to the debate on abortion, particularly as it relates to its legality, restriction, or permissibility. While some argue that life begins at conception, that is, life begins at fertilization, others say life begins at quickening, and some say at birth, and even argue that nobody knows when life begins until birth. The position one takes, would ultimately determine the person's value proposition on the ethical and legal considerations for abortion and if pregnancies are worthy of protection or otherwise.

The debate over 'when life begins' has shaped the various legislative policies on abortion in the United States. Quickening has been considered as a vital stage of pregnancy for determining that the fetus is a living being, in the sense that it is usually the moment a pregnant woman begins to feel the movement of her baby in her womb. In this regard, quickening is seen as the stage where the fetus becomes a living being. Thus, the fetus is a distinct living entity as soon as the woman begins to feel movement in her womb. At that point, the fetus ascends to the position of a human being which needs and deserves protection. The stance that life begins at conception is a further reflection of this view. Accordingly, States in the United States were influenced by this position whereat they enacted legislations which restricted abortions largely throughout the various stages of pregnancy, until these bans were lifted by the US Supreme Court in *Roe v. Wade*.[7]

[7] *Roe v. Wade* at page 5.

In *Roe v. Wade*, the Court was faced with the ultimate question of the living status of a fetus, and whether same is a person deserving of protection. In drawing the line between the legal status of a fetus or otherwise, the Court made recourse to the concept of conception, quickening, viability, and other theories in analyzing the debate about when a fetus becomes human. In the words of Mr. Justice Blackmun, who delivered the Opinion of the Court, he said:

> *"The [Hippocratic] Oath varies somewhat according to the particular translation, but in any translation the content is clear: 'I will give no deadly medicine to anyone if asked, nor suggest any such counsel; and in like manner I will not give to a woman a pessary to produce abortion,' or 'I will neither give a deadly drug to anybody if asked for it, nor will I make a suggestion to this effect. Similarly, I will not give to a woman an abortive remedy.' ...*
>
> *The Oath was not uncontested even in Hippocrates' day; only the Pythagorean school of philosophers frowned upon the related act of suicide....*
>
> *The Oath came to be popular. The emerging teachings of Christianity were in agreement with the Pythagorean ethic. The Oath 'became the nucleus of all medical ethics' and 'was applauded as the embodiment of truth.' .... it is 'a Pythagorean manifesto and not the expression of an absolute standard of medical conduct.'...*
>
> *It is undisputed that at common law, abortion performed before 'quickening' – the first recognizable movement of the fetus in utero, appearing usually from the 16th to the 18th week of pregnancy – was not an indictable offense. The absence of a common-law crime for pre-quickening abortion appears to have developed from a confluence of earlier philosophical, theological, and civil and canon law concepts of when life begins. These disciplines variously approached the question in terms of the point at which the embryo or fetus became 'formed' or recognizably human, or in terms of when a 'person' came into being, that is, infused with a 'soul' or 'animated.'..."*[8].

While the Court agreed that there were distinctions in the penalties for pre-quickened and post-quickened abortions, with the latter being more severe, the Court went on to opined that:

> *"It is thus apparent that at common law, at the time of the adoption of our Constitution, and throughout the major portion of the 19th century, abortion was viewed with less disfavor than under most American statutes currently in effect. Phrasing it another way, a woman enjoyed a substantially broader right to terminate a-pregnancy than she does in most States today. At least with respect to the early stage of pregnancy, and very possibly without such a limitation, the opportunity to make this choice was present in this country well into the 19th century. Even later, the law continued for some time to treat less punitively an abortion procured in early pregnancy."*[9]

The contention before the Court therefore was to decide whether States laws criminalizing abortions (particularly abortions in early pregnancies, that is prior to

[8] *Roe v. Wade* at pages 131–133.

[9] *Ibid*, pages 140–141.

the end of the first trimester), where made to protect the life of the pregnant woman rather than the preservation of prenatal life on the theory that life begins at conception. In resolving the debate, the Court then resorted to hold that a pregnant woman has a right to privacy, which is an inherent part of her right to liberty, and this right entitles her to decide the fate of her pregnancy, but within certain bounds. The Court stated as follows:

> *"This right of privacy, whether it be founded in the Fourteenth Amendment's concept of personal liberty and restrictions upon state action, as we feel it is, or, as the District Court determined, in the Ninth Amendment's reservation of rights to the people, is broad enough to encompass a woman's decision whether or not to terminate her pregnancy.... On the basis of elements such as these, appellant and some amici argue that the woman's right is absolute and that she is entitled to terminate her pregnancy at whatever time, in whatever way, and for whatever reason she alone chooses. With this we do not agree.... The Court's decisions recognizing a right of privacy also acknowledge that some state regulation in areas protected by that right is appropriate. As noted above, a State may properly assert important interests in safeguarding health, in maintaining medical standards, and in protecting potential life.... The privacy right involved, therefore, cannot be said to be absolute."*[10]

The Court could not define the "unborn" as a person as defined in the statutes, but it however considers it a "potential life" whose protection may outweigh that of the pregnant woman in certain circumstances, *albeit* at third trimester, as the woman's right to privacy in respect of abortion decisions is not absolute and must be measured against the interest of the State in preserving a potential life. The Court had this to say thus:

> *"We, therefore, conclude that the right of personal privacy includes the abortion decision, but that this right is not unqualified and must be considered against important state interests in regulation... As we have intimated above, it is reasonable and appropriate for a State to decide that at some point in time another interest, that of health of the mother or that of potential human life, becomes significantly involved. The woman's privacy is no longer sole and any right of privacy she possesses must be measured accordingly."*[11]

The Court though could not provide a definite answer to the question "when does life begin", but nevertheless was in agreement that life begins at some point during pregnancy for which the State would be justified to provide certain level of protection for the potential life. It added that the "compelling" point for which a State could regulate abortion is at viability, thus suggesting that life begins at viability. Here is what the Court opined:

> *"We need not resolve the difficult question of when life begins. When those trained in the respective disciplines of medicine, philosophy, and theology are unable to arrive at*

[10] *Ibid*, pages 153–154.
[11] *Ibid*, pages 154, 159.

any consensus, the judiciary, at this point in the development of man's knowledge, is not in a position to speculate as to the answer."[12]

On the whole, the court in resolving the matter against the State of Texas went on to say that:

"In view of all this, we do not agree that, by adopting one theory of life, Texas may override the rights of the pregnant woman that are at stake. We repeat, however, that the State does have an important and legitimate interest in preserving and protecting the health of the pregnant woman, whether she be a resident of the State or a nonresident who seeks medical consultation and treatment there, and that it has still another important and legitimate interest in protecting the potentiality of human life. These interests are separate and distinct. Each grows in substantiality as the woman approaches term and, at a point during pregnancy, each becomes 'compelling.'

With respect to the State's important and legitimate interest in the health of the mother, the "compelling" point, in the light of present medical knowledge, is at approximately the end of the first trimester.... It follows that, from and after this point, a State may regulate the abortion procedure to the extent that the regulation reasonably relates to the preservation and protection of maternal health.

With respect to the State's important and legitimate interest in potential life, the "compelling" point is at viability. This is so because the fetus then presumably has the capability of meaningful life outside the mother's womb. State regulation protective of fetal life after viability thus has both logical and biological justifications. If the State is interested in protecting fetal life after viability, it may go so far as to proscribe abortion during that period, except when it is necessary to preserve the life or health of the mother."[13]

In summary, the Court held as follows:

"(a) For the stage prior to approximately the end of the first trimester, the abortion decision and its effectuation must be left to the medical judgment of the pregnant woman's attending physician.

(b) For the stage subsequent to approximately the end of the first trimester, the State, in promoting its interest in the health of the mother, may, if it chooses, regulate the abortion procedure in ways that are reasonably related to maternal health.

(c) For the stage subsequent to viability, the State in promoting its interest in the potentiality of human life may, if it chooses, regulate, and even proscribe, abortion

[12] The Stoic believes that life begins at birth, while physicians and scientists are divided between the conception, life birth and viability (which appears to be the middle point). Some scholars hold the doctrine of "ensoulment" which can be traced to Aristotelian theory of "mediate animation." This view is though also found amongst some Christians, the Catholic Church on the other hand hold the view that life begins at conception, which view is also popular amongst many non-Catholics and physicians. *Roe v. Wade* at pages 159, 160–161.

[13] *Ibid*, pages 162–163. Viability according to the Court is usually placed at about 7 months (28 weeks) but that it may occur earlier, even at 24 weeks.

> *except where it is necessary, in appropriate medical judgment, for the preservation of the life or health of the mother."*[14]

In view of the above, the Court challenged and struck down in part Article 1196 of the Texas Penal Code in that case, which criminalizes abortion, on the grounds of vagueness, limiting its permissibility to only to save the life of the mother,[15] and without distinguishing between abortions procured in early pregnancy and those performed later. As such, the Court held that such code was unconstitutional as it is a violation of the Due Process Clause of the Fourteenth Amendment on the right to privacy and liberty.

Thus, a critical analysis of *Roe v. Wade* shows that the case did not give unfettered and absolute right to abortion. It however permitted same prior to viability, which could be between 24 to 28 weeks, thereafter the States can regulate or proscribe abortion for the sake of the unborn. In order words, the primary consideration must be that of the pregnant woman at any of the stages prior to viability and it is until viability, before consideration can be given to the potential life. A fetus is therefore considered viable where it can possibly exist outside the woman's womb, that is it can survive gestation and childbirth. In the US, viability is usually put around 24 weeks, although, the period of viability could differ between genders, race, and the statutory provisions on viability in the US differ from State to State.[16]

This decision gave room for US abortion laws across the country, whereby women could exercise their rights to abortion at various stages of pregnancies thereby asserting their reproductive rights in protection of their rights to autonomy, liberty, and equality. However, the decision in *Roe v. Wade* also propelled pro-life activists to challenge the position by redefining the beginning of life as conception for the purpose of protecting fetuses throughout pregnancy.

It is important to point out nonetheless the dissenting opinion of Mr. Justice Rehnquist in *Roe v. Wade* where he stated that the decision of the Court was given too broadly, as it addressed a hypothetical situation and further compounded by the introduction of the constitution rather than limiting the matter and the decision thereon to the set of facts presented to the Court. He posited that the decision imposes virtually no restrictions on medical abortions performed during the first trimester of pregnancy, whereas the Plaintiff who filed the case against the Texas statute was as at the date of the complaint may have been in her last trimester of pregnancy.[17]

In his opinion, the decision of the Court did not relate to the facts of the case in relation to the Plaintiff, but to the broader society as a whole, rather than the Plaintiff's own circumstances alone. He further argued that the regulation of abortion by the States did not violate any right of privacy, and that rights can be curtailed by due process of law. In his words:

---

[14] *Roe v. Wade*, page 165.

[15] See for example the case of *Rex v. Bourne* [1938] 3 All ER 615.

[16] Many States follow the federal standard of fetal viability which puts it between 23 and 24 weeks. However, Indiana, Iowa and Kansa have viability at 22 weeks, whereas some States like Nebraska put viability as early as 12 weeks. Also, girls are said to have higher survival rate to boys, which indicates that girls have lesser viability period than boys. As can be seen above, the definition of viability or identification of the period of viability could be fluid, and this position has changed the definition in *Roe v. Wade* which had defined viability as the period the fetus develops "the capability of meaningful life outside the mother's womb." See [3].

[17] *Ibid*, page 171.

> *"The decision here to break pregnancy into three distinct terms and to outline the permissible restrictions the State may impose in each one, for example, partakes more of judicial legislation than it does of a determination of the intent of the drafters of the Fourteenth Amendment. The fact that a majority of the States reflecting, after all, the majority sentiment in those States, have had restrictions on abortions for at least a century is a strong indication, it seems to me, that the asserted right to an abortion is not 'so rooted in the traditions and conscience of our people as to be ranked as fundamental,'"*[18]

The above dissenting position seems to have been justified by the decision in the recent case of *Dobbs v. Jackson Women's Health Organization*. The right to abortion came under intense scrutiny in *Dobbs v. Jackson*'s case, where the US Supreme Court had the opportunity to revisit its decision in the *Roe*'s case.

3. Overturning *Roe v. Wade*: a review of Dobbs v. Jackson Women's Health Organization

The case of *Roe v. Wade*[19] had over the years created heated debates on abortion between pro-abortionists and pro-life advocates. This case came under review by the US Supreme Court in *Dobbs v. Jackson Women's Health Organization* (*Dobbs'* case) (see [4]), wherein the court was faced with the question of whether "all pre-viability prohibitions on elective abortions are unconstitutional."

By way of a brief background, this case was instituted following the ban on most abortion operations after 15 weeks of conception by the State of Mississippi Gestational Age Act in 2018, which aims to protect the life of the unborn and provides that:

> *"Except in a medical emergency or in the case of a severe fetal abnormality, a person shall not intentionally or knowingly perform ... or induce an abortion of an unborn human being if the probable gestational age of the unborn human being has been determined to be greater than fifteen (15) weeks."*[20]

The respondent, an abortion clinic, sued the State's health officer, Thomas E. Dobbs, challenging the constitutionality of the ban on the ground that it violates the constitutional right to abortion as established in the cases of *Roe v. Wade*[21] and *Planned Parenthood v. Casey.*[22] The challenge to the Act was upheld by the District Court which stated that the ban was a violation of the US Constitution and precedents which prohibit States from placing a ban on pre-viability abortion. This position was affirmed by the Fifth Circuit and then appealed to the Supreme Court by way of certiorari.

---

[18] *Ibid*, page 174.

[19] The decision in *Roe v. Wade* struck down federal and States laws against abortion on the basis of the Due Process Clause of the Fourteenth Amendment to the United States Constitution, which was adopted in 9 July 1868 as one of the Reconstruction Amendments.

[20] § 4(b). §3(f) of the Act defines "gestational age" to be "the age of an unborn human being as calculated from the first day of the last menstrual period of the pregnant woman."

[21] See note 19.

[22] The decision was based on the women's right to privacy as guaranteeing their right to abortion. See note 2.

The Supreme Court recognized that abortion was a critical moral issue for which the Court needed to provide direction. In the words of Mr. Justice Alito in delivering the Opinion of the Court held:[23]

> *"Abortion presents a profound moral issue on which Americans hold sharply conflicting views. Some believe fervently that a human person comes into being at conception and that abortion ends an innocent life. Others feel just as strongly that any regulation of abortion invades a woman's right to control her own body and prevents women from achieving full equality. Still others in a third group think that abortion should be allowed under some but not all circumstances, and those within this group hold a variety of views about the particular restrictions that should be imposed."*[24]

It was argued at the Supreme Court that the Mississippi Gestational Age Act was constitutional on the basis that it satisfies the rational-basis review and that the case of *Roe v. Wade* was wrongly decided and should be overruled. The Supreme Court in deciding the *Dobbs'* case effectively overturned the long-standing precedent established by the landmark cases of *Roe v. Wade* and *Planned Parenthood v. Casey* in holding that the Constitution of the United States does not confer a right to abortion, and further that the Constitution does not forbid the States from regulating or prohibiting abortion and as such the authority to regulate or prohibit abortion is returned to the people and their elected representatives.

The rationales for the decision of the Court are that there is no express provision in the Constitution or its amendments granting a right to obtain abortion; the right to abortion is not rooted in the history and tradition of United States as it is not an essential component of America's "scheme of ordered liberty";[25] and that the right to obtain abortion cannot be justified as forming part of the entrenched rights supported by other precedents. Further, the Court took the view that the critical moral problem generated by abortion had not been a focus of prior precedents, and as such cannot constitute a basis for supporting a right to abortion. In the words of the Court, it stated as follows:

> *"We hold that Roe and Casey must be overruled. The Constitution makes no reference to abortion, and no such right is implicitly protected by any constitutional provision, including the one on which the defenders of Roe and Casey now chiefly rely—the Due Process Clause of the Fourteenth Amendment. That provision has been held to guarantee some rights that are not mentioned in the Constitution, but any such right must be 'deeply rooted in this Nation's history and tradition' and 'implicit in the concept of ordered liberty.' Washington v. Glucksberg, 521 U. S. 702, 721 (1997).*

[23] The *Dobbs'* Opinion was written by Associate Justice Samuel Alito. Associate Justices Clarence Thomas, Neil M. Gorsuch, Brett M. Kavanaugh, and Amy Coney Barrett joined the opinion. Thomas and Kavanaugh filed concurring opinions. Chief Justice John Roberts filed an opinion concurring in the judgment. Associate Justices Stephen Breyer, Sonia Sotomayor, and Elena Kagan dissented.

[24] *Dobbs v. Jackson Women's Health Organization (supra)*, at page 1.

[25] That is no State in the United States had any constitutional provision that recognized the right to abortion and there was no such support for the right to obtain abortion in American law until few years before *Roe v. Wade* in the latter part of the twentieth century. Prior to *Roe v. Wade*, abortion at any stage of the pregnancy was a crime in three quarter of American States. Contra, *Planned Parenthood v. Casey (supra)* and *Roe v. Wade (supra)*.

> *The right to abortion does not fall within this category....*
>
> *It is time to heed the Constitution and return the issue of abortion to the people's elected representatives. 'The permissibility of abortion, and the limitations, upon it, are to be resolved like most important questions in our democracy: by citizens trying to persuade one another and then voting.' Casey, 505 U. S., at 979. That is what the Constitution and the rule of law demand."*

Thus, *Dobb's* has reversed the federal right to abortion, and has provided the States the power to regulate abortion at any stage or otherwise. In other words, the exercise of the "right to abortion" must be circumscribed within the permissible limits of the States legislations. This decision has been greeted with mixed feelings of resentment from pro-abortionists and jubilation from pro-lifers.

4. Differing views on the decision of the supreme court

Many, particularly pro-choice activists, have attacked the judgment of the Court as a retrogressive move. Some have alleged that the decision was initiated, pushed forward, and supported by centrist-conservative justices appointed by Republican Presidents George W.H. Bush and Donald Trump, who now form the majority of justices at the Supreme Court, because all three appointed justices by Democrat Presidents Bill Clinton and Barak Obama dissented. They argued that the right to abortion was an extension and integral part of the broader prescribed rights which includes the right to privacy as recognized in *Roe v. Wade* and right to liberty, which is the freedom to make "intimate and personal choices" which are "central to personal dignity and autonomy" as held in *Planned Parenthood v. Casey*.[26]

For example, President Joe Biden had described the decision of the Supreme Court as "cruel", stating that it "is the culmination of a deliberate effort over decades to upset the balance of our law. It's the realization of an extreme ideology and a tragic error by the Supreme Court, in my view"[27] and urged the Congress to codify *Roe v. Wade* into federal law. In the words of the Vice President, Kamala Harris she said:

> *"This is the first time in the history of our nation that a constitutional right has been taken from the people of America. And what is that right? — some might ask. It's the right to privacy.*
>
> *Think about it as the right for each person to make intimate decisions about heart and home; decisions about the right to start a family, including contraception, such as IUDs and the morning-after pill; decisions about whether to have a child...; decisions to marry the person you love — Obergefell v. Hodges, Loving vs. Virginia...*
>
> *In holding that it is not deeply rooted in our history, today's decision on that theory, then, calls into question other rights that we thought were settled, such as the right to use birth control, the right to same-sex marriage, the right to interracial marriage...*

[26] See the Syllabus on the Judgment of the Court in *Dobbs v. Jackson Women's Health Organization* No. 19–1392, at page 3.

[27] https://www.catholicnewsagency.com/news/251630/biden-calls-dobbs-decision-a-tragic-error-calls-on-congress-to-codify-abortion-rights.

> *Today, I invite all people to stand together in defense of one of the most fundamental ideals and principles that for generations, for centuries, I believe, we have held dear, which is that fundamental principle about the importance of liberty — to stand for liberty, to stand for freedom, to stand for self-determination, and for the right to privacy."*[28]

Pro-life proponents have also added their voices in the commentaries on the decision of the Court. One of whom is the former president of the United States, Donald Trump. He praised the decision of the Court and said it "is following the Constitution, and giving rights back when they should have been given long ago."[29] The U.S. Conference of Catholic Bishops (USCCB) has expressed overwhelming acceptance of the decision stating that:

> *"America was founded on the truth that all men and women are created equal, with God-given rights to life, liberty, and the pursuit of happiness...*
>
> *This truth was grievously denied by the U.S. Supreme Court's Roe v. Wade ruling, which legalized and normalized the taking of innocent human life...*
>
> *We thank God today that the Court has now overturned this decision."*

While the debate on the decision of the Supreme Court continues, it is important to briefly highlights some reservations the American people have held about the decision and the likely impact it could have on the American society.

5. Implications on the American society

In *Roe*'s case the Court agreed that there was no absolute right to abortion. It however, provided conditions for exercise of the right to abortion viz-a-viz States' intervention on the ground of "compelling State interest". For a pregnancy within the first trimester, the pregnant woman has unrestricted right to determine whether to terminate or keep it and the State cannot regulate such. However, for pregnancies within the second and third trimesters, the State may regulate but must do so for the protection of the pregnant woman in the former instance, and then the unborn child in the latter case, except the life of the mother is at risk. Thus, the States cannot regulate abortion for the protection of the unborn at any stage until the third trimester.

At the stage of the third trimester, the potential life would have become viable, and being capable of living outside the body of the mother, the Court opined that such unborn could be afforded some level of legal protection. Hence, the decision of the Court in *Roe*'s case provided room for unregulated medical abortions up to the point of viability, which in most cases, starts at third trimester. In addition, the discretion of the States to regulate or not for protection of the unborn at third trimester seems to have offered an opportunity for an unlimited period for abortion.

Americans had since *Roe*'s case championed the idea of women's right to abortion, but this has also faced criticisms from pro-life groups. It was only until recently, the

---

[28] See https://www.whitehouse.gov/briefing-room/speeches-remarks/2022/06/24/remarks-by-vice-president-harris-on-the-supreme-court-decision-to-overturn-roe-v-wade/.

[29] See https://www.foxnews.com/politics/trump-praises-supreme-court-decision-overturning-roe-v-wade.

Supreme Court once again revisited the debate on abortion and made a review on the *Roe*'s case. Unsurprisingly, since the Court handed down its decision in *Dobbs*' case, the American society had expressed anxieties over what could be the implications of the decision on other matters on human rights, particularly those in relation to liberty and privacy.

The *Dobbs*' case has presented a new dimension to the issues of human rights, morality, public policies, and administration justice. Against this background matters relating to right to contraceptives, rights of LGBTQI+, amongst others, had come to fore. Thus, many Americans have expressed fear that some of these previously settled rights could then be challenged on the basis of *Dobbs.* Consequently, it is feared that the legal precedents of *Lawrence v. Texas,*[30] *United States v. Windsor,*[31] *Hollingsworth v. Perry*[32] and *Obergefell v. Hodges,*[33] recognizing the right to privacy and right to marry for same-sex couple as guaranteed by the Due Process Clause and Equal Protection Clause of the Fourteenth Amendment to the American Constitution, and other rights available to LGBTQI+ community, may come under question and threats as a result of the overturn of *Roe v. Wade*. Suffice to say that the decision in *Dobbs*' case could create a precedent for many other controversial legal, social, moral cum religious issues in the near future.

This uncertainty by the American public is fuelled by the view that some justices of the US Supreme Court are centrist-conservative, and specifically Catholic justices who would hardly be able to separate their Christian beliefs from the doctrines of law. However, this fear may be considered imaginative than realistic as the Court had emphasized that its decision only relates to the constitutional rights to obtain abortion and no other rights. Hence, an expression of anxiety over threats to other rights would seem to be unsubstantiated.

Further, apart from the fear of threat to other rights, there are also anxieties in relation to the direction of States across the United States in their various legislations on the differing definition of a viable foetus. The Mississippi's Gestational Age Act, which was the subject of controversy in the *Dobbs*' case seems to have put the age of "viability" at 15 weeks.[34] In Alabama and Arkansas, for example, abortion at conception is outlawed and only permitted in exceptional circumstances for life and physical health.

In Missouri abortion is prohibited after 8 weeks of pregnancy, while in some States like Georgia, Ohio, South Carolina and Tennessee, 6 weeks is prescribed, in Idaho, 22 weeks is statutorily prescribed and in some other States it is 18 to 20 weeks.[35] Virginia however imposes a statutory limit on abortion in the 3rd trimester of pregnancy which usually begins at 27 weeks, whereas in California, New York, Delaware, Washington, Connecticut and some others, a foetal viability

[30] 539 U.S. 558 (2003).

[31] 570 U.S. 744 (2013).

[32] 570 U.S. 693 (2013) (Docket No. 12-144).

[33] 576 U.S. 644 (2015).

[34] See Mississippi Code Annotated § 41–41–191(4)(b) (2018), which defines a foetus as an "unborn human being."

[35] Though these laws were initially enjoined by court orders and has not taken effect, with the decision in *Dobbs*' case, these States can then take appropriate steps to enforce the laws.

standard is imposed as the gestational age limit for abortion following the federal standard of foetal viability.

The decision in *Dobbs* has also brought to the forefront the legal consideration for frozen embryos and whether same can qualify as human beings or persons capable of protection. An embryo and a fetus both refer to a baby but at different stages of development. Thus, an embryo is a fertilized egg, and the developing zygote is considered an embryo from the moment of conception (fertilization) till about the eight or ninth week of gestation, where it thereafter becomes a fetus. In this regard, an embryo is a potential human being. What then happens if the embryo is frozen? Considering that the decision in *Dobb's* case, does not imply that frozen embryos are persons, it does not however rule out the potentiality of frozen embryo becoming a human person. Hence, States' laws which prohibit abortion at the point of fertilization,[36] could also be extended as legal protection for frozen embryos.

Prior to *Dobb* there was no likely liability for "wrongful death" of lost embryos unlike loss of post-viable fetus. However, "after *Dobbs*, liability risks could attach for any damage to embryos in transporting or receiving from one clinic to the other, or if spilling culture media in the lab and losing several embryos or if there is active decision making on the part of an individual or couple to discard the embryo. Added to this is the complexity of insurance coverage for everything from medical malpractice to criminal abandonment" [5, 6].

Thus, the questions of who a child is, and whether an unborn child is a human being that has a constitutional guaranteed right to life may continue to be subject of debate or legislations in time to come, and this could influence a review of some of these States' laws in future.

6. Conclusion

The decision of the US Supreme Court which overturns *Roe v. Wade* does not necessarily ban or criminalize abortion nor does it recognize the constitutional right to life for an unborn child. It does however take away the encoded legal restrictions created by the judiciary which prevent States across the United States from restricting or prohibiting abortion, especially pre-viability abortions. *Dobbs'* decision will uncontrovertibly have a long-time impact on the American society, the judicial system, policy formulation and administration in many years to come.

The power to restrict, prohibit or otherwise allow abortion is now left in the hands of the States, and the outcome of the exercise of this power by the various component States will be seen in the coming days. While the *Dobbs'* case is an unprecedented legal victory for the pro-life movement and a loss for pro-choice, the debates on abortion right and the right to life of an unborn child remain continuing controversial argument which are yet to be over.

---

[36] See Abolition of Abortion in Louisiana Act of 2022 (H.B. 813, 2022 Leg.). This law bans abortion at any stage of development irrespective of viability. The law, which was previously enjoined, took full effect following the decision of the Supreme Court in *Dobbs v. Jackson*. See also Oklahoma House Bill 4327.

Author details

Richmond Ekhosuehi Idaeho
Jackson, Etti and Edu, Victoria Island, Lagos, Nigeria

*Address all correspondence to: richmondidaeho7@gmail.com

References

[1] United Nations. 2023. Available from: https://www.un.org/en/global-issues/human-rights#:~:text=Human%20rights%20are%20rights%20inherent,and%20education%2C%20and%20many%20more [Accessed: June 23, 2023]

[2] Jacobs SA. Biologists' consensus on 'when life begins'. In: SSRN. 2018. Available from: http://papers.ssrn.com/paper.taf?abstract_id=3211703

[3] Stacey M. What is fetal viability, and how does it impact abortion cases?. Available from: https://www.wthr.com/article/news/health/fetal-viability-explained/531-c39665b1-1bcd-46d3-88be-4620894b23a5#:~:text=In%20the%20deciding%20opinion%20for,Roe%20v [Accessed: June 23, 2023]

[4] Idaeho RE. Turning Point in American Abortion Law: US Supreme Court's Reversal of *Roe V. Wade*. 2022. Available at SSRN: https://ssrn.com/abstract=4158561

[5] Letterie G, Fox D. Legal personhood and frozen embryos: Implications for fertility patients and providers in Post-Roe America. Journal of Law and the Biosciences. January-June 2023;**10**(1):7. Available from: https://www.ncbi.nlm.nih.gov/pmc/articles/PMC10200124/#fn44 [Accessed: June 26, 2023]

[6] Kawwass JF et al. Embryo donation: National trends and outcomes, 2000-2013. American Journal of Obstetrics Gynecology. 2016;**215**:747. Available from: https://pubmed.ncbi.nlm.nih.gov/27393270/

Chapter 4

Femicide: A Forensic View

Jennifer Garcia Ospina and Patricia Eugenia Diaz Montoya

Abstract

Femicide, understood as the death of a woman, because of her status as a woman o because of her gender identity, represents a challenge from the forensic approach, which requires a critical look from the medical examiner to interpret the findings he sees in the corpses and integrate it with the context information provided by authority, in such a way that a complete and comprehensive autopsy is carried out that guides the authorities in the judicial investigation process. This chapter seeks to take a look at those aspects of the autopsy that allow a comprehensive approach to death with suspected femicide.

Keywords: femicide, violence against women, human rights violations, forensics, autopsy

1. Introduction

Feminicide, understood as the death of a woman, because of her status as a woman or because of her gender identity [1], is already a recognized public health problem, in addition to a serious violation of human rights, and although it is not yet known its magnitude in the world, given the methodological difficulties in differentiating these murders from other homicides of women [2], the latest United Nations report on homicides [3] estimates that in 2012, 92,766 women were murdered and 47% of these murders were occurred by the couple or the family, being the seventh cause of premature death in women in the world.

In United States, alone the rates have fluctuated between 3.8–4.5 deaths per 100,000 women [4]. In Canada, a woman is murdered every 2.5 days — ranging from 144 to 178 murders each year between 2015 and 2019 and in 2021, of the women murdered, 50% were killed by intimate partners and 26% by family members [5]. In Pakistan, the exact figure is yet to be known but according to an estimate thousands of women are victims of dowry deaths. Moreover, nearly 500 women a year are the victims of honor killings [6].

Domestic abuse and femicide rates are particularly high in Latin America [7], a region with the second-highest female homicide rate in the world, second only to Africa [8].

In Colombia (**Figure 1**), femicides maintain a constant trend over time, in 2019 from 1001 homicides of women, 109 cases were femicides (10.88%); in 2020, 989 homicides of women were committed, of which 90 cases were femicides (9.1%), in 2021 of the 978 registered homicides of women, 106 were femicides (10.83%) and during the first quarter of 2022 of 264 registered homicides, 26 cases correspond to femicides (9.84%) [9]. In our population, the majority of deaths are caused by

IntechOpen

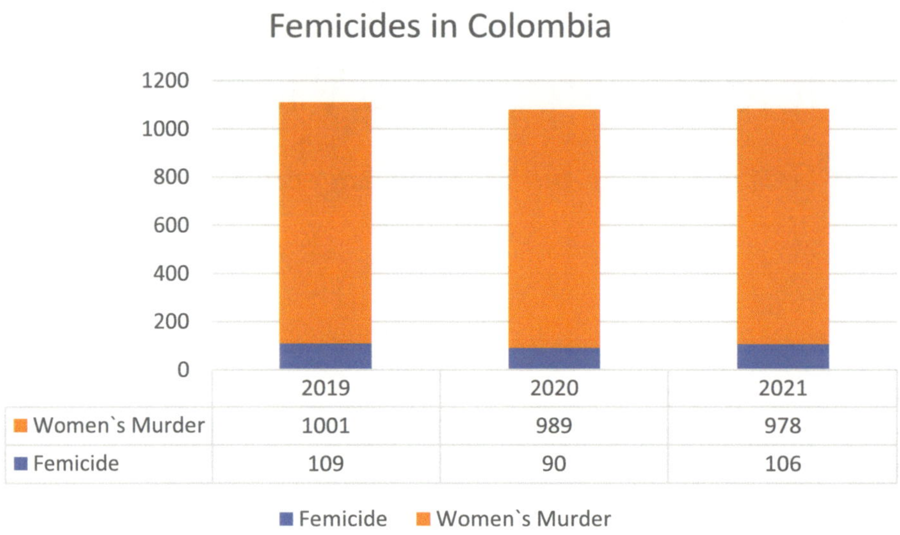

Figure 1.
Femicides in Colombia.

firearm projectiles and stab trauma, primarily affecting women between 29 and 59 years of age [9].

For medical examiners, the medico-legal approach to femicide represents a challenge that requires a holistic and integrative view to interpret the findings on the body and analyze them together with the contextual information, in such a way that a complete and comprehensive autopsy is carried out that guide the authorities in judicial investigation processes. This chapter seeks to take a look at those aspects of the autopsy that allow a comprehensive approach to deaths with suspected femicide.

2. Autopsy for suspected cases of femicide

The medical-forensic investigation of corpses whose death raises suspicions of femicide is not broadly different from the approach that should be carried out in cases where human rights violations are suspected [10]. In technical terms, the autopsy examination must follow the usual steps, beginning with the examination of the site where the body was found, continuing with the autopsy itself and ending with the complementary examinations necessary for each case [11].

3. Examination of the body discovery site

In some countries, coroners regularly attend crime scene as part of their forensic work; in Colombia, medical examiners do not have judicial police functions, that is, legally we are not empowered to process the crime scene, instead, the scenes are processed by technical staff of the CTI (judicial investigation technical body) or SIJIN (Judicial Investigation Section) who through a document known as Technical Inspection Report, where they provide all the information from the scene to medical examiners so he can proceed to perform the autopsy. In that order of ideas, it is essential that medical examiners carry out a complete analysis of the information provided prior to the start of the autopsy, including the evaluation of the photographs from the scene and details of the discovery of the corpse such as position, location, elements on and around it, clothing arrangement, blood dripping patterns and other elements from the scene that guide specific procedures and searches during the autopsy process. If the information available in relation to the scene and finding of the body is limited or insufficient, it is recommended to carry out all the necessary steps to obtain it, prior to the start of the autopsy. Likewise, it is highly relevant to have a complete context as possible in relation to the circumstances surrounding the events, in order to be able to differentiate between femicide and homicide, it is crucial to establish the elements that motivated the aggressor's conduct [12], hence the context analysis is essential to establish a medical-legal approach to the forensic diagnosis of femicide [13] and guide the procedures, evidence and other actions within the autopsy process. Therefore, it is recommended that the investigation of femicide cases be carried out from a gender perspective with inter-institutional work geared and coupled in order to find the elements associated with criminal motivation and obtain efficient results in the judicial investigation process [11].

4. Autopsy

In all cases, a complete autopsy should be performed, including opening of the cranial and thoracoabdominal cavity with systematic dissection of the visceral block and organ-by-organ dissection [11]. Although the expert is free to choose the order in which the body is going to intervene as long as he does not omit performing procedures, it is recommended in these cases to carry out the external and internal examination with a systematic cephalocaudal order.

External examination: A thorough and detailed inspection of the body and the container or packaging in which the body was brought to the autopsy room must be carried out. The use of forensic lights is ideal [11], however, given the limitation of the resource, the use of magnifying glasses is advisable to magnify the visual field of the evaluator. After reviewing the packaging and recovering the evidence found it in a pertinent manner, proceed with the analysis of the body. Check the scalp for the presence of abrasions, ecchymoses, bruises, or areas of traumatic alopecia. Check the face, eyes, conjunctivae, ears, nose and oral cavity. Look for the presence of petechiae in the conjunctiva or oral mucosa that may be associated with asphyxia or hypoxic phenomena, rule out the presence of soft tissue trauma, especially in the nostrils and labial or peri-oral mucosa that may be associated with suffocation [14].

Rule out the presence of hidden trauma to the ears, with an otoscope (in cases where the context suggests the possibility of torture), check the tympanic membrane and rule out ruptures. Evaluate the oral cavity very well looking at the state of the teeth, the presence of trauma to the tongue, hemorrhages in the braces and in cases where an associated sexual offense is suspected, take the pertinent smears, including the interdental smear with dental floss. For the revision of the neck, it is always recommended to do it in hyperextension, ruling out the presence of grooves, bruises or abrasions that may be related to asphyxia maneuvers such as hanging/strangulation [14]. In the thorax and abdomen, rule out the presence of trauma, sugilations (especially in the breasts) and adequately document the findings according to their nature. The genital examination must be complete, initially inspecting the external part of the vagina, anus and inner thighs, looking for the presence of fluids, abrasions, bruises or sugilations. Evaluate the hymen indicating its shape, elasticity and the presence or absence of tears [15]. Check the anus to identify the presence or absence of tears and tone [15]. In the extremities, attention should be paid to any pattern of injury that indicates fight or defense and the nails and nail beds should be checked very well with recovery of trace evidence and nail clipping in cases that warrant it.

If the context suggests the possibility of an associated sexual offense and/or a corpse is observed in a sexualized position, with clothes improperly placed or naked (without a logical explanation for its nudity) with pattern injuries consistent with bites or sugilations and stains or whitish fluids to the human eye or orange under forensic lights, it is recommended to carry out a detailed sexological examination before washing the corpse and to document the morphology of the traumatic injuries [15, 16]. This sexological examination includes the evaluation of the garments, ideally with forensic lights looking for the presence of fluids (blood different from the victim, semen, saliva) or trace evidence from the aggressor that allow establishing a causal link between the victim and the aggressor in accordance with the Locard principle. Swabs should be taken from the oral cavity, breasts, vagina and anus [16]. Likewise, if fluids suggestive of saliva or semen are identified on the corpse by forensic lights, take smears of said areas [16].

If trauma by firearm or trauma by knife is evident in the corpse, the proper guidelines for dealing with this type of case must be followed, in Colombia the approach is oriented according to the guide: Deaths due to injuries by firearm projectile [17] and the guide of deaths due to Injuries by sharp weapon [18].

In cases of stab trauma, especially throat slitting or extensive soft tissue trauma, it is recommended to perform wound reconstruction (**Figure 2**) [14], in order to assess their morphology and guide the number, type, extent and trajectory of the injuries.

Particularly important is the search, documentation and interpretation of injury patterns related to death, such as [11]:

- *Overkill*: The number of injuries is more than necessary to cause death, it can occur both in cases of knife and firearm, the finding injuries in different stages of vitality is characteristic, which indicates that even after being dead, the person continued to be the object of aggression [11].

- *Defeminization*: Corresponds to depersonalization maneuvers that aim to destroy those characteristics associated with femininity, including injuries, mutilations or amputations of female organs (genitals, breasts), facial disfigurement, haircuts and even nail removal [11].

- *Dismemberment*: maneuver to reduce the body to fragments, which can be carried out for various reasons such as transporting the body from the primary scene, preventing the identification of the deceased, sending a message or even being the causal mechanism of death [19].

- *Defense wounds* [18]: These are related to wounds that, due to their cutting mechanism and their location mainly on the extremities, suggest a fight or defense by the victim during the aggression.

Internal examination: Perform bimastoid incision and lift the scalp, evaluating the presence of subgaleal hematomas. Remove the muscular plane and the galea to

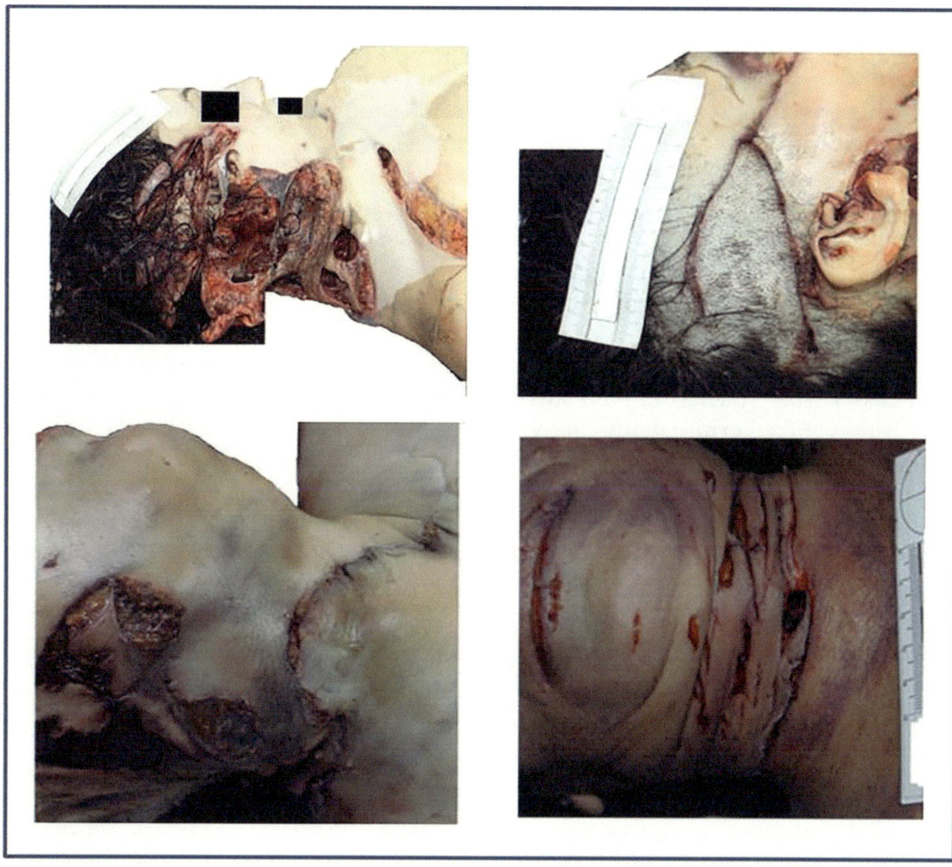

Figure 2.
Reconstruction of injuries caused with a blunt object (machete). Own source.

evaluate the skull bones and rule out the presence of fractures, proceed with the opening of the cranial vault, with extraction of the brain and a detailed review of it, seeking to rule out any type of trauma [11]. Do not forget to review and photographically document the base of the skull. After emptying the neck vessels after exploring the head, proceed with the anterior neck dissection and facial lift, seeking to document or rule out the presence of hematomas and/or fractures of the laryngeal, thyroid, and hyoid cartilages. The foregoing for cases in which asphyxiating maneuvers such as strangulation or hanging are particularly suspected [14]. If hyoid fractures are found and if radiographs are available, it is recommended to carry out radiological documentation of the fracture (**Figure 3**) [14].

Proceed with the internal examination of the thoracic and abdominal cavity plane by plane with extraction of the visceral block, inspection and section of each organ. In cases where an associated sexual offense is suspected, carry out a special dissection of the pelvic block with a smear of the rectal mucosa, cervix and uterine cavity. If the context is suggestive of cruel and inhuman treatment or torture, apply all the recommendations mentioned in the Minnesota protocol [20]. Always keep in mind the practice of additional special procedures in cases that require it [11]:

- Exploration by anatomical planes of the face: In all cases where facial injuries are documented or suspected. Special emphasis is placed on femicides associated with domestic violence, femicides associated with organized crime, femicides within the context of war and armed conflict, and femicides with evidence or suspicion of related sexual activity (**Figure 4**).

- Exploration by anatomical planes of the neck: In all cases in which injuries are suspected or evidenced at the cervical level; asphyxia due to neck compression, penetrating firearm projectile wounds to the neck, penetrating stab wounds to the neck, blunt force trauma to the neck (**Figure 5**).

- Examination by anatomical planes of the back extended to the extremities: In all cases where back trauma is suspected. Special emphasis: femicides associated with organized crime, femicides within the context of war and armed conflict (**Figure 6**).

- Extraction of complete female genitalia: Where traumatic injuries are suspected at the level of internal genital organs. Particularly important in femicides with suspected related sexual activity (**Figure 7**).

Finally, it should be kept in mind that the entire procedure must be accompanied by adequate and sequential photographic documentation [11, 20] of both the positive findings and the absence of relevant findings that allow hypotheses related to the cause of death to be ruled out.

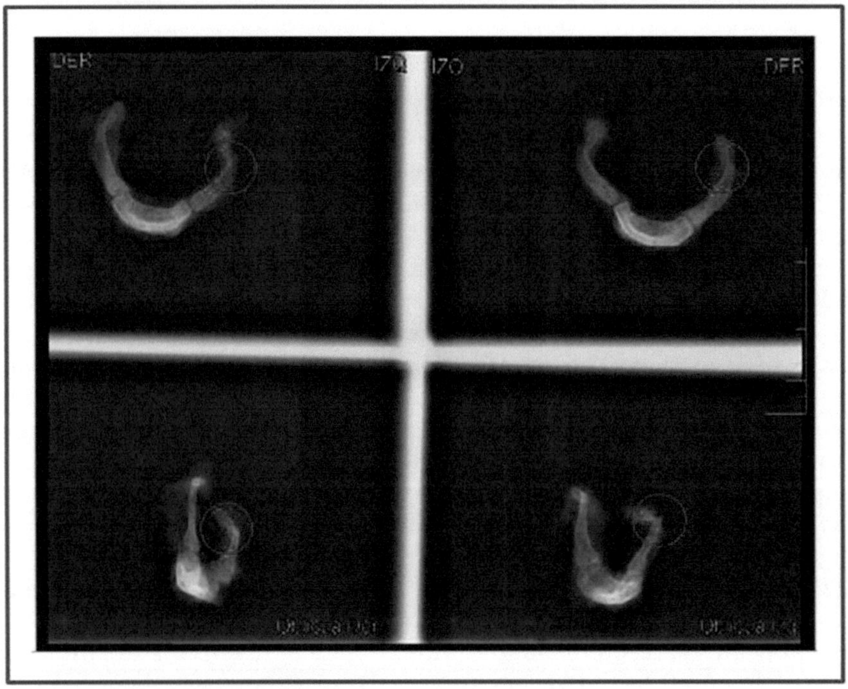

Figure 3.
Fracture of the left lateral horn of the hyoid bone in a case of strangulation. Own source.

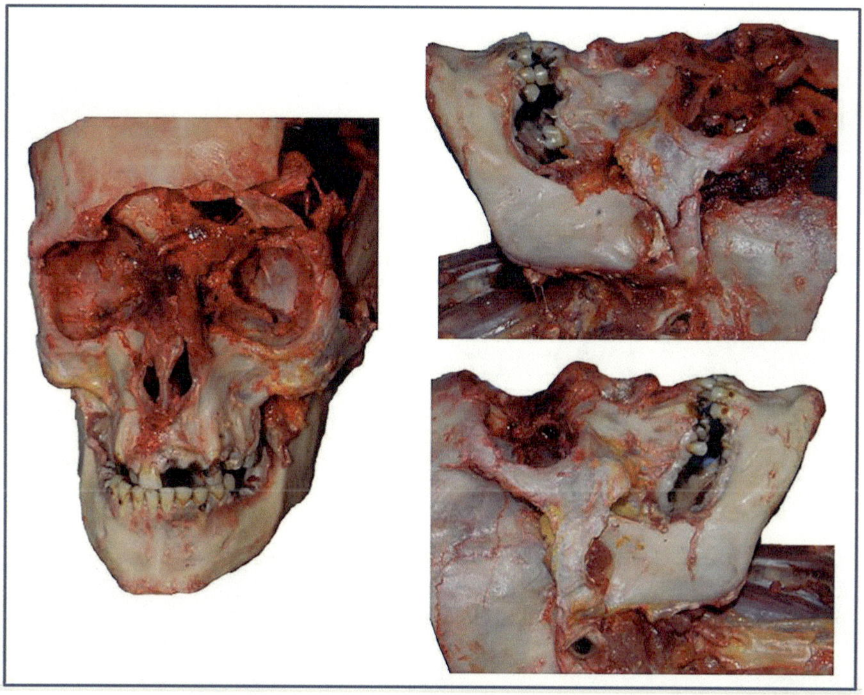

Figure 4.
Special dissection with complete facial lifting, in which comminuted fracture in the frontal region and linear fracture in the left zygomatic bone can be seen. Own source.

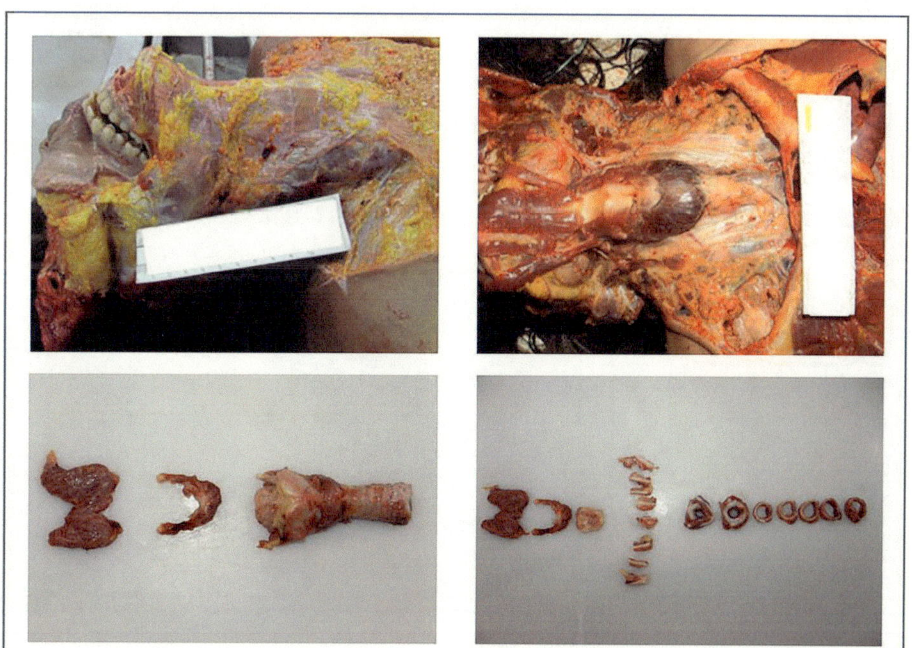

Figure 5.
Special anterior neck dissection by anatomical planes with laryngeal cartilage dissection. Own source.

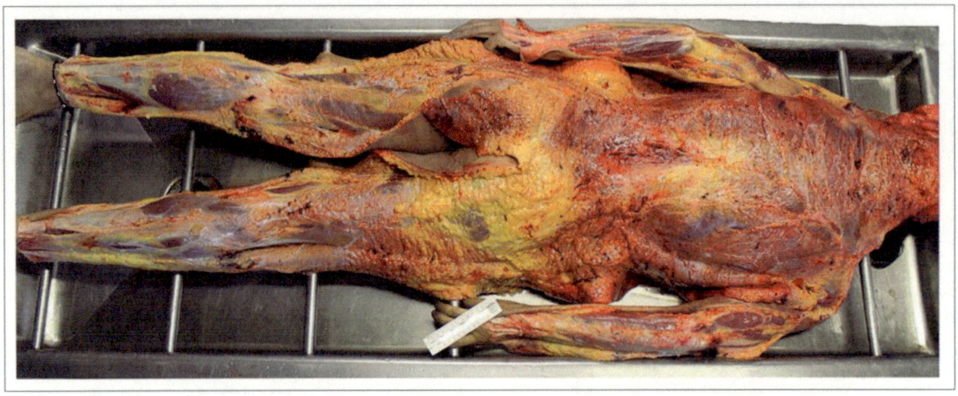

Figure 6.
Posterior special dissection in elongated X, which seeks to reveal the presence or absence of occult trauma. Own source.

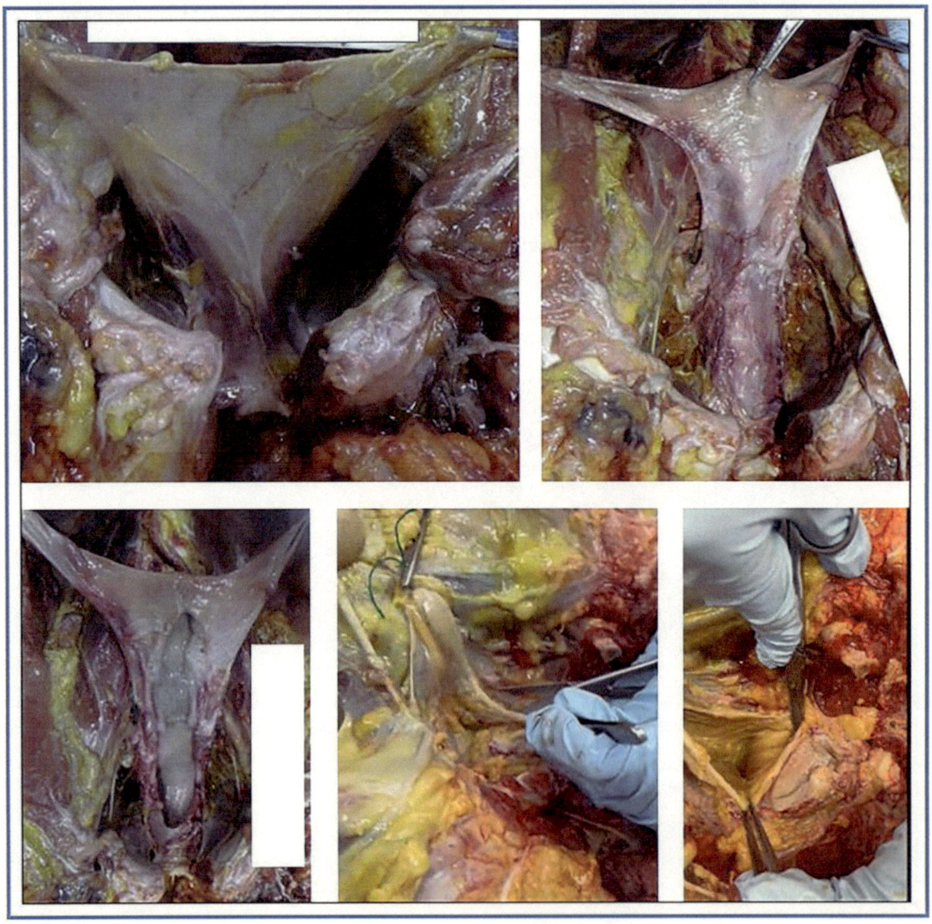

Figure 7.
Special dissection of the female pelvic block, in which the bladder, the uterus and vaginal cavity, and the rectum are successively illustrated. Indicated in cases of deaths with suspected associated sexual crime. It is recommended to take smears of the cervix, uterine cavity and rectal mucosa during the dissection. Own source.

5. Complementary tests

The type of samples recovered and the tests requested will depend on the context of the case and the state of the body [11], however, the possibility of obtaining matrices suitable for toxicological analysis and samples for biology must always be guaranteed, especially if there is an associated sexual offense. Regarding the matrices for toxicological examination, it will always be ideal to recover blood and urine, however, other matrices such as vitreous humor, bile, gastric content, bladder lavage, CSF, liver, kidney, muscle, purging fluid, among others, can also be considered, among others; the selection of one or another matrix will finally be limited to the state of the corpse and the demonstrative capacity according to the context of the case [11]. In firearm cases, it is imperative to recover all possible ballistic evidence [17] (weapons, projectiles, pellets, projectile sleeves, clothing, among others) and seek the respective processing in the corresponding laboratory. In cases of stabbing [18], if the traumatic element is found, seek detailed photographic documentation of it, as well as the determination of its dimensions and guarantee the fingerprint search, as well as the genetic examination looking for different profiles from that of the victim. For cases of strangulation, gagging and forced immobilization, if constrictor elements are available, remember the possibility of analysis looking for the epithelial cells of the aggressor [21]. In cases of dismemberment, corpses abandoned inside plastic containers or suffocation with a bag, keep in mind the possibility of looking for fingerprints on these materials [20]. In relation to the garments, their analysis includes a detailed description that ranges from their position on the body to the type, brand, color, material, size and presence of any fluid, tear or damage that calls the attention of the evaluator [17, 18]. It is advisable to use forensic lights for the analysis of garments, however, if the resource is not available, remember to use a magnifying glass, in order to carry out a more detailed and thorough analysis. As for X-Rays, their use will depend on the availability of the resource. If available, it is particularly useful in cases of firearm projectiles, decomposed, burned or calcined, skeletonized and throat-cut corpses [11]. Histopathology is very useful to document the dating of lesions or pathophysiological processes associated with the mechanism of death when there are periods of survival after trauma [11].

Regarding the autopsy expert report, in analysis and conclusion [11] sections, it is important to carry out an interpretation of the findings integrated with the analysis of the context where not only the cause and manner of death are sought to be clarified, but it is also highly relevant to guide to the authority on the type of femicide and the presence or absence of circumstantial elements that guide precautionary measures by the aggressor or punitive aggravating factors associated with the victim, such as pregnancy, age under 18 year old, inability to resist or states of helplessness associated with substance use or forced immobilization, physical disability and associated sexual assault, among others.

Author details

Jennifer Garcia Ospina and Patricia Eugenia Diaz Montoya*
National Institute of Legal Medicine and Forensic Science in Medellin, Colombia

*Address all correspondence to: pediaz@medicinalegal.gov.co

References

[1] Law. Congress of Colombia. Criminal Type of Femicide as an Autonomous Crime. Law Rosa Elvira Celis. 2015 July 6;**19**:49565

[2] Sanz-Barbero B, Otero-Garcia L, Boira S, Marcuello C, Cases CV. COST Action Femicide Across Europe, a transnational cooperation space for the study and approach to feminicide in Europe. Gac Sanitation. 2016;**30**(5):393-396

[3] Gibbons J, editor. Global Study on Homicide 2013. Vienna: United Nations Office on Drugs and Crime; 2014. p. 166

[4] Garcia-Moreno C. Gender inequality and fire-related deaths in India. The Lancet. 2009;**373**:1230-1231

[5] Nori L, Bradley MD. The physician's role in the prevention of femicide in Canada. CMAJ. 2021;**193**:E1844-E1845

[6] Nasrullah M, Haggi S, Cummings KJ. The epidemiological patterns of honor killing of women in Pakistan. European Journal of Public Health. 2009;**19**: 193-197

[7] Alvarez-Garavito C, Acosta-González HN. Femicide in Latin America: An economic approach. Development and Society Magazine. 2021. DOI: 10.13043/DYS.88.1

[8] World Health Organization. World Health Statistics 2013. Colombia: World Health Organization; 2013

[9] National Institute of Legal Medicine and Forensic Sciences. Observatory of violence. External cause injuries in Colombia. Available from: https://www.medicinalegal.gov.co/cifras-de-lesiones-de-causa-externa

[10] López Hernández E, Peña Rodríguez D, Salas Ramírez KM. Basic Guidelines and Minimum Contents for the Elaboration of a Model Protocol for the Investigation of Femicides/Feminicides. Mexico: Regional Alliance for women's access to justice; 2012

[11] National Institute of Legal Medicine and Forensic Sciences. Guide of recommendations for the judicial investigation, attention and prevention of deaths with suspicion of femicide. 2016

[12] Constitutional Court of Colombia. Judgment C – 539 of 2016. 2016. https://www.corteconstitucional.gov.co/relatoria/2016/C-539-16.htm

[13] Jennifer Garcia Ospina. Characterization of Homicide and Variables Associated with Femicide. Spain: Spanish Academic Publisher; 2019

[14] Tellez NR. Forensic Pathology, an Approach Focused on Human Rights. Colombia: National University of Colombia; 2014

[15] National Institute of Legal Medicine and Forensic Sciences. Guide for a comprehensive forensic approach in the investigation of sexual violence. Colombia. 2018. http://www.medicinalegal.gov.co

[16] National Institute of Legal Medicine and Forensic Sciences. The medical-legal autopsy in victims of forced disappearance: Documentation of torture and sexual violence. Available from: http://www.medicinalegal.gov.co

[17] National Institute of Legal Medicine and Forensic Sciences. Guide to deaths due to firearm projectile injuries.

2014. Available from: http://www.medicinalegal.gov.co

[18] National Institute of Legal Medicine and Forensic Sciences. Guide to deaths due to stab wounds. 2014. Available from: http://www.medicinalegal.gov.co

[19] Guarín CV, Ospina JG, Castaño CFM. Factors associated with the identification of quartered or dismembered bodies in Medellin, (Colombia). Rev Esp Med Legal. 2020. DOI: 10.1016/j.reml.2019.12.001

[20] United Nations Organization. UN Manual for the prevention and effective investigation of summary, extrajudicial and arbitrary and legal executions. 1991. AN. DOC. E/ST/SCDHA/12.1991. Available from: http://www.hchr.org.co/publicaciones/libros/Protocolo%20de%20Minesota.pdf

[21] National Institute of Legal Medicine and Forensic Sciences. Guide of recommendations for the forensic approach in cases where torture or other cruel, inhuman or degrading treatment or punishment is investigated or suspected. 2014. Available from: http://www.medicinalegal.gov.co

Section 2

Ethical Perspectives

Chapter 5

Ethical Controversy Surrounding the Revision of the Uniform Determination of Death Act in the United States

Osamu Muramoto

Abstract

This chapter reviews fundamental ethical controversy surrounding the ongoing effort to revise the Uniform Determination of Death Act in the United States. Instead of focusing on the process of the revision itself, the chapter explores the underlying ethical debate over brain death that has been ongoing for many decades and finally culminated in this revision. Three issues are focused: the requirement for consent and personal exemptions before applying brain death for the diagnosis of death; redefining the areas of the brain that have ceased to function in the definition of brain death; and codifying the American Academy of Neurology as the authority to issue the standards of the diagnosis of brain death. The chapter concludes that allowing the personal choice of death determination gives a pragmatic compromise to the disputed definition and practice of diagnosing brain death. So long as all risks and imperfections of the diagnosis are accepted through the consenting process, there is nothing ethically objectionable to continuing the current practice of diagnosing brain death as a successful tool to facilitate heart-beating organ donation without violating the dead-donor rule. By contrast, precluding personal choice and imposing legal restrictions to consent and exemptions would further erode public trust.

Keywords: brain death, uniform determination of death act, informed consent, conscientious objection, organ donation

1. Introduction

> *"An individual who has sustained either (1) irreversible cessation of circulatory and respiratory functions, or (2) irreversible cessation of all functions of the entire brain, including the brain stem, is dead. A determination of death must be made in accordance with accepted medical standards" (The Uniform Determination of Death Act 1981).*

The Uniform Determination of Death Act (UDDA—as quoted above) is, as of middle 2023, under review by the Uniform Law Commission (ULC) for revision.

The uniform laws in the United States are meant to be a non-binding model law, which can guide each state to legislate its statutes [1]. The current UDDA was drafted by the President's Commission for the Study of Ethical Problems in Medicine and Biomedical and Behavioral Research and approved by the ULC in 1981. Subsequently, 36 states, the District of Columbia, and the US Virgin Islands have adopted the UDDA. The remaining states have enacted similar legislation or court decision [2]. While the concept of brain death was introduced in the 1950s and '60s as an irreversible coma [3], the UDDA formally codified this concept throughout the United States. The UDDA has been pivotal since its adoption to guide medical practice in neurocritical care and organ transplantation. Below the surface of this "uniformity" of the acceptance of the UDDA, however, it has been rigged by vigorous and persistent controversies and genuine and sound disagreement from the beginning [4]. From the standpoint of bioethics, this controversy itself has always been a major area of ethical deliberation, but what has made this controversy further more challenging is the fact that brain death has been successfully integrated into clinical practice. Without this practice, heart-beating organ donation would have been almost impossible, and the intensive care unit would have been overcrowded with patients whose disposition is uncertain. This stark contrast between clinical success and unresolved ethical disagreement makes this debate on the definition of death so entangled.

The purpose of this chapter is not to update the ongoing effort to revise the UDDA. The revision should have been completed by the time this chapter is read. Moreover, it is entirely unclear how many states are willing to enact the revised UDDA. It is possible that the issues taken up in this revision will continue to be debated at state levels. Instead of focusing on this short-term development, this chapter concentrates on the ethical analysis of three focal points that triggered the current revision: (1) persistent functioning of the hypothalamus despite the requirement of the cessation of all functions of the entire brain; (2) specific professional organizations are designated as the sole authority for the standards of the diagnosis of brain death; and (3) notification to the next to kin and consent is required to initiate the evaluation for brain death [5]. While these points have emerged recently in medical-legal cases, underlying ethical issues that culminated in them have been debated for decades. The main focus of this chapter is those fundamental ethical controversies underlying the current revision of the UDDA. Of particular, the third item, consent and related issue of exemption, is most pertinent to clinical ethics, and this will be discussed in detail.

The plan of this chapter is as follows. The next section discusses the controversy surrounding the consent and exemption for diagnosing brain death. The issue is not just a narrow procedural question, even if the ULC might leave it to state levels if they view it as a relatively minor point. The fundamental ethical issue underlying the consent and exemption about diagnosing brain death is the personal choice of how we die, or death is determined. It is at the core of end-of-life ethics. The third section discusses the problem of brain regions being included for irreversible cessation. The fourth section discusses the possible revision to add specific medical organizations as the sole authority of the protocol for diagnosing brain death. While these two sections deal with some technical issues, there are also important ethical concerns. The final section will concisely present overall moral viewpoints of this long-standing controversy over brain death, which is just rekindled by the revision of the UDDA, and final thoughts for a pragmatic solution.

2. The ethical controversy over the consent and exemption of brain death

2.1 Background of consent and exemption about brain death

The overarching concept of consent and exemption is the personal choice regarding brain death. Should individuals be allowed to choose whether they are diagnosed and declared dead by neurologic criteria? Some commentators, notably Veatch, Ross, and others [6, 7], have long advocated personal choice among three definitions of death: circulatory, whole-brain, and higher-brain. They have argued that personal choice of the definition of death should be legally permitted. However, the higher-brain definition has never gathered broad support. It defines irreversible coma, or persistent vegetative state (PVS), as death. However, there are many technical difficulties: First, the diagnosis of PVS or the irreversibility of coma is notoriously inaccurate, with up to 40% of diagnoses turning out to be errors. Moreover, even when the diagnosis is correct, up to 24 percent of cases regain consciousness in 2 years. Although functional imaging tests have been used to increase the accuracy of diagnosis and prognosis, no reliable data is available for the rate of false positives in long-term follow-up [6]. Although Veatch and Ross continue to favor the higher-brain definition, they acknowledge that it is not a feasible option until we know more about how to diagnose irreversible coma without false positives. Therefore, we will focus on the first two definitions. Moreover, since circulatory death has been the traditional definition and is still by far the most widely used one, it is the default definition unless brain death is used. For this reason, we will only focus on whether there should be any personal choice to avoid using brain death as the definition of death (and by default, circulatory death is chosen).

2.2 Argument for personal choice

In this section, we will examine common reasons that personal choice for brain death—through exemption or consent—is desirable. So far, personal choice is not admitted to the use of neurologic criteria for death diagnosis except for several states where exemption is possible: New Jersey [8], New York [9], California [10], and Illinois [11]. All mention religion as the reason for exemption, consideration, or accommodation in using neurologic criteria to remove life support. California also mentions cultural practices and New York mentions moral objection. Before going into the details of exemption and consent, let us consider why personal choice is desirable. In general, the current trend in clinical medicine is to accommodate patients' preferences so long as it does not create secondary problems, such as violating others' rights and excessive resource allocation. That is precisely why patients generally prefer "personalized" medicine and informed consent or decline in almost every aspect of clinical medicine. Of course, the diagnosis and definition of death are quite different from other therapies and diagnoses. However, the question is whether there are specific reasons for excepting death diagnosis and what is common and different from other therapies and diagnoses.

The final moment of human life is profoundly personal, spiritual, and valued. How a person is judged to have expired and classified as deceased is a moral value judgment. As Veatch and Ross appropriately pointed out [6], no matter how precisely neurological criteria identify an irreversibly non-functional brain and how many reasons are given that a body without a functioning brain is equivalent to a dead body, neurology or any other knowledge of medical science cannot and should not determine that the person who possesses that brain is alive or dead. That judgment is entirely one of value, answered by each person's moral, philosophical, and religious convictions. Death is fundamentally a process, not a momentary event [12]. It is only made to appear a moment for the convenience of the law and society. If there is room for personal choice for such a moment, society and the law should accommodate it. Of course, that does not mean that anyone can arbitrarily decide the moment of their death. We already have a universal and indisputable moment of death since immemorial: death by circulatory criteria. It is a sudden departure introduced by brain death from this time-honored tradition over the past several decades that triggered all these challenges. This discord is not necessarily from certain cultural, religious, or philosophical traditions but the tradition of the entire humanity. It is only a matter of fundamental morality to accommodate such a value choice in our multi-cultural, value-diverse, and democratic society, as opposed to suppressing any diverse values through "physician power" [13].

2.3 Argument for consent before applying the neurologic criteria of death

It is unclear at this time whether the personal choice for the definition and diagnosis of death is considered by the ULC morally important in our society. If they consider it important enough, the ULC might incorporate personal choice as an exemption because several states have already implemented it. Regarding consent, the current proposal is only about its rejection, stating that "consent is not required to initiate an evaluation [of death by neurologic criteria]" [5]. Such a clause has already been adopted by the state legislature in Nevada [14]. Whether the revised UDDA would incorporate these points or leave it to state decisions is unclear. Regardless, let us consider using informed consent before diagnosing brain death because informed consent is primarily a matter of medical ethics, and the law plays a role when a legal dispute arises.

From the viewpoint of the proponent of informed consent before performing the diagnostic procedure of brain death, it is plain that informed consent is required as much as any other medical procedure of similar importance [15]. Needless to say, informed consent is used in almost every aspect of clinical medicine today, as long as the intervention involves any risk or significant consequences to patients. Consent is not limited to physical and mental risk but the risk of diagnostic errors, the consequences of false positives and negatives, and the setback of personal interest.

Obviously, most patients and families want to avoid a false-positive diagnosis of death or classifying a living patient as dead. Compared to other diagnostic tests, knowing the risk of false positives is paramount. They will likely require their physicians to rule it out completely. In this regard, three critical pieces of information must be disclosed to the family before the diagnostic protocol of brain death is initiated. First, unlike other diagnostic tests, we do not have well-controlled clinical trials to accurately evaluate the rate of false positives and negatives of the diagnosis of brain death. This lack of definitive data is because almost every case of brain death is disposed of promptly after the diagnosis, either by terminating life-support or removing vital organs for transplantation. There have been anecdotal rare cases that were kept on life support, such as pregnant women and those cases whose families insisted on life support. There has been no systematic study to repeat the diagnostic test for brain death in intervals to see if the diagnosis is reproducible. Second, repeated reports of violating established diagnostic protocols [16–18] implicate procedural risks. Additionally, there are several reported cases of diagnostic errors [19, 20].

As with other medical procedures, the procedural risk of the apnea test, which is crucial to diagnosing brain death, is an indispensable part of informed consent. The apnea test induces hypercapnia by stopping the ventilator after full oxygen saturation. Hypercapnia triggers the respiratory drive if the brainstem is still functioning. If there is no respiratory movement in the chest and abdomen, the test is positive and consistent with brain death. The risk comes mainly from the fact that hypercapnia can raise intracranial pressure, which is part of the causative pathophysiology of brain death [21]. The test can further aggravate already elevated intracranial pressure, perpetuating the underlying pathophysiology of brain death. It also causes hypotension and arrhythmia, which could be fatal.

The risk from the apnea test may indeed be small, but it is not negligible. Many very low-risk diagnostic procedures, such as treadmill exercise tests and lumbar puncture, are routinely done with informed consent. The magnitude of risk is always compared to the benefit of the procedure. It is this relative magnitude of the risk versus benefit that decides whether the procedure is acceptable or not. As long as the apnea test involves greater than zero risk, it has to be compared to the zero benefits of the apnea test for most patients. For them, this risk/benefit ratio becomes infinitely large. It is also true that the diagnosis of brain death could be beneficial if the patient is known to have the wish to become a heart-beating organ donor. This fact can be ascertained, and the risk/benefit ratio is estimated during the conference for informed consent *only before* the procedure.[1]

2.4 Argument against informed consent before initiating the diagnostic procedure of brain death

Opponents of the consent requirement, who proposed to state explicitly that consent is not required in the proposed revised UDDA [5], give several reasons. According to Lewis and Pope, (1) consent will limit "physicians' power to determine death," (2) "inciting families to seek injunctions to continue organ support after brain death," and (3) "forcing hospitals to dispense valuable resources such as ventilators, beds, medications, and clinician time, to dead patients" [13]. In a separate paper, Lewis, Bonnie, and Pope [22] give the following four reasons: "[Requiring consent would] (1) challenge the integrity of DNC [death by neurologic criteria]; (2) increase the number of objections to DNC; (3) necessitate allocation of health care money and resources to patients who may be dead in lieu of those who are alive; and (4) create a double standard for death determination, given that consent is not required for determination of death by cardiopulmonary criteria."

These points can be grouped under three headings: (1) Integrity argument, or the challenge to physician's unrestricted "power to determine death"; (2) Symmetry argument, or consent requirement has to be the same for brain death and circulatory death; and (3) Utilitarian argument, or consent requirement will prolong the hospital stay and incite family's objections by delaying the diagnosis of brain death and consume more resources. In what follows, we will examine each of these three objections.

---

[1] Information provided before informed consent does not necessarily have to be comprehensive, but because the risk is misdiagnosing life as death, the standards can be the highest for some patients. Also, some families may forego informed consent due to poor prognosis, and as with other informed consent, patients have every right to waver informed consent at any time and for any reason.

2.4.1 Integrity argument

This argument stems from a typical confusion and conflation between declaring death, which is a legal procedure and diagnosing the state of the brain as brain death, which is a medical procedure. It is true that the legal declaration of death follows the medical diagnosis of death in usual circumstances, but not always. The most well-known example is when the patient is pregnant. A physician may medically diagnose brain death but may not legally determine that the patient is dead. Nor does the law require physicians to declare death immediately after the diagnosis of death. If that were the case, all dying patients would have to be admitted to the ICU to avoid missing the moment they die. But, of course, it is absurd, and many patients die at home, and a physician declares death probably the following day. It is left to the discretion of physicians when they make a diagnosis of death. Informed consent is entirely about the medical diagnosis and has no force over the legal determination of death. Only after the diagnosis of death has been made does the legal duty to issue a death certificate starts. Consent or refusal does not directly affect the "physician's power" to legally determine death. A physician has full power to declare death whenever necessary information becomes available for death. If the patient declines the test for brain death, the physician still has the full power to declare death when the patient's heart stops irreversibly.

The revised state law of Nevada [14] states, "brain death determination is a clinical decision that does not require the consent of the person's authorized representative or the family member with the authority to consent or withhold consent." It is unclear why "a clinical decision" does not require consent when other numerous clinical decisions routinely require consent, including a clinical decision as simple as removing a wart. The ULC should be astute enough to spot this logical flaw.

2.4.2 Symmetry argument

The argument claims that because consent is not required for the diagnosis of circulatory death, neither should it be for the diagnosis of brain death. There are several problems in this argument. First, it is incomprehensible why two different practices must be symmetrical in consent requirements. The diagnosis of circulatory death and brain death is indeed the diagnosis of death. But that does not entail that the consent requirement must be the same. There is no logical or practical reason for this symmetry. This argument is equivalent to demanding the same consent requirement for a colonoscopy and a stool blood test because they both diagnose colon cancer. It is false because a colonoscopy involves much more risk than a stool blood test even when they diagnose the same condition.

Second, this argument neglects the fundamental reason a certain intervention does not require consent. Besides the risk of intervention, as already discussed above, the presence of an alternative is critical. If there is no alternative to an intervention, consent is moot. Almost every medical intervention has an alternative: no intervention. The diagnosis of circulatory death is a rare exception: no alternative. Everybody acknowledges that someone has undergone circulatory death when they do. The body becomes cold and rigid, followed by putrefaction. Nobody can ignore this reality. There is no qualm that the permanent cessation of the heart and breathing is the exceptionless human destiny.

The opponents of the consent requirement want to argue that brain death also comes with no alternative. But of course, unlike circulatory death determination and like any other medical intervention, a valid alternative for diagnosing brain death exists: not to do it. No intervention means not proceeding to the diagnostic procedure of brain death and continuing life support, waiting for circulatory death unless the condition improves, preparing for non-heart-beating organ donation if the patient is a qualified donor, or transitioning to palliative care. They also neglect that circulatory death sometimes requires consent. When a do-not-resuscitate (DNR) order is placed, circulatory death is diagnosed without confirming its irreversibility. In this case, there are clear risks (the heart could still be restarted if resuscitation was done) and an alternative (trying to restart the heart). Consent for this protocol of diagnosing circulatory death makes perfect sense exactly because there are risks and alternatives. It is false to claim that circulatory death is always diagnosed without consent.

2.4.3 Utilitarian argument

As quoted above, the opponents of the consent requirement have argued that consent would "necessitate allocation of health care money and resources to patients who may be dead in lieu of those who are alive" [22]. It is true that the sooner we diagnose a patient dead, the more we can spare healthcare resources. Should we reallocate resources from "patients who may be dead" to those who are alive by diagnosing death sooner than later? What is problematic about this apparently correct argument? Nobody would disagree that it is important to spare medical resources and refrain from wasting them. However, it would be controversial to do so by diagnosing someone as dead hurriedly when the family has no idea why the patient is dead before the heart stops. The family wants to have a death diagnosis later than sooner. By definition, circulatory death never precedes brain death. It is logical for an unprepared family to choose circulatory death, which is the latest and default death. It is against the fundamental moral principle of clinical medicine to ignore such a basic human desire to delay the death of the loved one maximally. We cannot arbitrarily test every near-death patient for death so that we would not miss the earliest chance to vacate ICU beds. Our primary duty is to continue life-saving treatment, particularly if the patient and/or family are not ready for death diagnosis without clear signs of death. Cost saving without balancing with serious ethical consideration is a recipe for bureaucratic health care.

Of course, that does not mean we must continue futile treatment indefinitely. There is a better way to conserve resources than unilaterally classifying a patient dead: transitioning to comfort care after a full agreement with the family. By doing so, there is no need to allocate the ICU resources and physician time to make an extra effort to make an unnecessary and risky diagnosis of brain death. Known organ donors are, of course, exceptions. If the patient is considered a heart-beating donor, diagnosing brain death could be beneficial to achieve his or her known wishes. There are no qualms about proceeding to the diagnosis of brain death. However, for most other cases, particularly when the patient is known to decline organ donation, it would be wasteful to test for brain death. Such patients are best handled with palliative care followed by the determination of death by circulatory criteria if further treatments are deemed ineffective.

What about "inciting families to seek injunctions to continue organ support after brain death," which is one of the reasons not to offer consent, as quoted above? When we review those families who were "incited" and sought legal injunctions to continue organ support, such incitement was triggered *not* by well-conducted informed consent but by the *lack* thereof. In fact, there has been no informed consent before brain death determination in those cases known from the court record. Consent was *never* the reason for inciting those families that took their cases to court. On the contrary, unilateral declaration of death by neurologic criteria without any agreement is the reason. Those cases are more of the reason that we need to explain in detail what entails brain death diagnosis, and all questions are answered before proceeding to the procedure.

Additionally, such disagreement about death determination often comes from those families in cultural, religious, and racial minorities who hold different values from the dominant social groups of the United States, such as many physicians and lawyers who are highly educated and belong to a higher socioeconomic class than those families. Instead of compassionately understanding their values and seeking common grounds through a conference for informed consent, those opponents of consent treat them simply as "incited families" and try to override them by "physician power." Even when informed consent was not required, more compassionate and sincere communication before a brain death diagnosis might have averted such legal actions.

2.5 Argument for exemption from applying the neurologic criteria of death

Most proponents of personal choice for the definition of death, such as Veatch [6], have focused their argument not on informed consent but on the legal exemption from applying the neurologic criteria for death determination. In such arguments, the public is encouraged to decide in advance how death is determined so that this advance directive is honored when death comes. As mentioned in 2.2, four states, New Jersey, New York, California, and Illinois, provide exemption, consideration, or accommodation based on religious, cultural, or moral reasons. Exemptions are not in the proposed revision of the UDDA, but since they are already incorporated in several state laws, the ULC might incorporate them into the revised UDDA.

Before brain death was introduced, such diverse differences in death judgment among different traditions were rare. This was because circulatory death is mostly transparent and uniform with few and rare exceptions. There is little room for disagreement regarding death determination by circulatory criteria. Brain death is entirely different. The diagnosis of brain death and the determination of death by neurologic criteria are so removed from the transparency that unless the family and surrogate blindly trust the words of physicians, acceptance of death at the sight of numerous signs of life is an enormous challenge. Policy- and lawmakers may or may not consider the diversity of values, but certainly, a significant portion of the population would raise concern about treating a person whose brain is non-functional as dead if they knew the reality of the state of a brain-dead person. It is this diversity of values in this multicultural, multi-ethnic society of the United States that makes value-based exemptions much more important than in smaller and more homogeneous countries.

2.5.1 Argument for religious and cultural exemptions

The religious exemption has a special place in the United States due to the First Amendment of the US Constitution that separates the church and state. Under this special treatment of religion, it is often difficult to legally enforce some decisions, particularly those related to personal medical decisions, against religious beliefs. For example, the traditional Jewish view is that death occurs upon the separation of the soul from the body. Some Jews accept only irreversible cardiopulmonary cessation as the definition of death. On the other hand, religion exceptionalism may be viewed as discrimination against non-religious people. Moreover, religion is notoriously difficult to define because it is inherently a cluster concept without sharp demarcation from non-religion. Religiosity is often a matter of degree. It needs to be clarified how a state defines religious objection and how it is determined and implemented. Is it necessary for a person to belong to a specific religious organization, or is occasional affiliation sufficient? Some people are raised in the family or culture of a certain religion. Is that enough to consider an objection from such people religious? Given such potential challenges surrounding the treatment of religion in uniform ways, an introduction of sweeping religious exemption may not be an ideal solution. Again, in our value-diverse society, a broader conception of the value-based objection, including moral, philosophical, conscientious, as well as religious objection, seems more desirable.

2.5.2 Argument for non-religious exemptions

In contemporary secular society, giving privileged status to any decision framed as "religious" became more controversial when the same privilege is denied if the decision is framed as non-religious. Aforesaid, California mentions cultural practices as a reason to "make reasonable efforts to accommodate"; New York mentions moral objection as the reason for "reasonable accommodation to the determination." No state mentions philosophical reason or, more broadly, personal reason. That means that no state under the current UDDA will consider any objection based on a personal belief that brain death is not that person's death.[2] Or suppose someone questions the sensitivity, specificity, and safety of the procedure of brain death diagnosis, or on the grounds of simple and basic risk-benefit analysis in medicine, and wants to opt out of such a death determination. In that case, there is no recourse for exemption from death determination by brain death. That is why Veatch and Ross [6] advocate all-encompassing conscientious clause or conscientious objection, as opposed to religious, cultural, or philosophical exemption.

2.5.3 Argument against exemptions from neurologic criteria of death

The same objections against consent can also apply to exemption. Many cases of extended somatic survival, such as Jahi McMath [23], invoked religious exemption in New Jersey. As long as the cost of sustaining somatic life is funded by health care insurance, which is the case in New Jersey, the utilitarian argument can also apply to exemptions. On the other hand, since exemptions are often invoked after the diagnosis is made, the integrity argument and symmetry argument against consent may not apply to exemption. Moreover, since religion has a special status in the US Constitution, opponents of consent do not voice their opposition to religious exemption, at least in the same tenor and rigor.

While this is not exactly the opposition, several practical and technical difficulties are involved in exemptions. First, how many of the general population would bother to register their preferences regarding the definition of death when brain death is

[2] Brain death is deeply rooted in the Cartesian mind-body dualism that says that the thinking mind is the essence of being a human. Euroamerican centrism in philosophy tends to forget that this belief is only one species of metaphysical views among many others in the world.

relatively rare and often unimaginable? When only one-third of the population uses advance directives (AD) for end-of-life care [24], how much more is it unlikely that they think seriously about the definition of death? Brain death can happen regardless of age, for example, due to sudden subarachnoid hemorrhage, devastating brain trauma, drowning, and complications from surgical procedures. That means it is likely that brain death happens in a population without established AD. For this reason, it is further more difficult to register such a choice in advance before such an unexpected and rare event falls upon them.

Second, as many empirical studies indicate, the general public does not adequately understand the meaning and significance of brain death [25]. It is not uncommon that they confuse brain death with a coma and (persistent) vegetative state, such as Terri Schiavo. Laypeople (and most likely even many physicians) cannot differentiate between coma, vegetative state, brain death, and even locked-in syndrome by viewing bedside appearances of photos and video clips of those patients.[3] With this level of general understanding of brain death, how can medical professionals rely on an AD of a patient regarding their preference for the definition of death? Third, as a well-known problem of AD, there are always difficulties finding such directives on time when brain death becomes rapidly imminent. Such an exemption status is only known through well-informed family members or other surrogate decision-makers who are familiar with the AD.

And lastly, it is unclear whether exemptions are also applied to minors. Those state laws do not say explicitly about minors. This is probably because the minor's religious commitment is not reliable enough to grant a religious exemption. As often seen in cases of Jehovah's Witness parents who refuse blood transfusions for their children, parental religious exemptions are often overridden by the court. It is unclear about the definition of death, but if New Jersey is any guide, unlike cases of Jehovah's Witnesses, parental religious exemptions are granted for their children.

2.6 Exemption versus consent

The above contrast between exemption and consent has several important implications. First, informed consent is not a ceremony of signing paperwork. Informed consent is a process of bidirectional information exchange and frank dialog between the medical team and the family or surrogate to reach a common ground or shared decision-making. Exemption never comes with such a deliberative process between the family and medical team. If informed consent is done correctly, the resulting shared decision is based on precise information on the patient's medical condition. It also reflects the particular preferences of the patient and the family facing the patient's imminent death.

These patients have several options, depending on the patient's condition and the availability of appropriate medical programs. First, as long as the patient is an organ donor, the diagnostic protocol for brain death can be started in a timely manner to fulfill the patient's wishes to donate vital organs. If the patient is not deemed a heart-beating donor, they could still receive medical treatment with an expectant observation for spontaneous improvement, though this is uncommon as long as the patient is judged in imminent brain death. Once the family agrees that the prognosis is extremely poor regardless of brain death or not, transitioning to palliative care and eventually withdrawing life support is an important option. Of course, it is also

[3] For an up-to-date review of changing classifications of the disorders of consciousness and other conditions that mimic brain death, refer to Kondziella and Stevens [26].

common that patients who miss the diagnosis of brain death for various reasons soon succumb to circulatory death. For those not candidates for heart-beating donation, a donation after circulatory determination of death without diagnosing brain death can also be discussed before transitioning to palliative care.

These are not abstract decisions on exempting from brain death in advance and are expressed in AD without any specific information regarding the context of the medical events and alternative choices. In contrast, religious exemptions and accommodations in current state statutes mostly refer to a special treatment regarding the timing of the removal of life support *after* the diagnosis of brain death. Of course, some religious exemptions, such as those of the orthodox Jewish community in New Jersey, are well known to local medical providers, and in such special situations, the entire process of diagnosing brain death may be exempted. In most other cases of religious and conscientious exemptions and accommodations, brain death is already diagnosed, but death is not legally declared, and life-supporting treatment continues. This fact is crucial for the utilitarian argument. Since consent or decline takes place before the diagnosis of brain death, it is improbable that those cases that decline brain death end up with a very long process of somatic support. They have several alternatives to brain death. In contrast, religious exemption cases, such as Jahi McMath case, have only one option: indefinitely continue life-support until cardiac arrest. Moreover, consent can achieve the purpose of exemptions and conscientious objections in most cases. Even if exemption status is unknown at the time of acute brain injury, and AD has not been established or located on time, consent can cover all the needs of exemptions and AD, as long as the surrogates properly execute their roles and decline consent.

From the viewpoint of the value of individual choice in medical care, and death determination in particular, all instruments are desirable, including AD with conscientious objection clauses and religious and cultural exemptions. Informed consent or decline immediately before the diagnostic procedure can ensure that the stated choice of these instruments is respected. However, it is unlikely that these will be incorporated into the revised UDDA. A likely scenario is to read that "consent is not required to initiate an evaluation" as given in the proposed revision [5]. If so, the issue of personal choice could be discussed at the level of state legislators.

Nevertheless, that does not mean the family cannot request informed consent. This proposed revision does not say that consent is prohibited. That means that the family may still request consent. If this happens, can the medical team refuse consent? It is an important open question in clinical ethics. Consent is not legally required, but what about a moral requirement, particularly if the family explicitly requests it? The law does not directly dictate most informed consent in clinical settings. Medical ethics primarily covers it. Depending on how the revision is worded and state laws are amended, medical ethicists might face the question of whether the medical team can refuse consent when the family requests it. Ethicists in Nevada might start seeing such cases since Nevada is so far the only state that explicitly mentions in the state law that consent is not required.

3. The controversy over the anatomic regions of the non-functional brain

3.1 The hypothalamic functions in brain death

The possible revision of the brain region pertains to a long-standing debate about whether "the cessation of the all functions of the entire brain" is indeed a necessary and sufficient condition of human death. There are three categories of challenges. The first is that human death is only the irreversible cessation of circulatory and respiratory functions (the first definition of the UDDA), the second is the irreversible cessation of all functions of the entire brain (the second definition of the UDDA), and the third is the cessation of so-called the higher brain. As mentioned in 2.1, the higher brain definition has minimal support and is not considered for this revision. The debate continues, but by the legal authority of the UDDA, the whole brain criteria have been accepted for brain death, while the overwhelming majority of the population die from circulatory death. However, recent legal cases and case reports increasingly challenged the whole brain criteria because it became clearer that there are important areas of the brain that are not entirely non-functional in cases of brain death. Particularly at issue is the hypothalamus. Michael Nair-Collins group [27, 28] provided an extensive literature review, demonstrating that this part of the brain often survives brain death and continues functioning.

The hypothalamus is only a small part of the brain but has many integrative functions that are indispensable not only for the brain function but for the vital functions of the whole body. The hypothalamus controls the energy metabolism, fluid and electrolyte balance, thermoregulation (including fever responses), and the homeostasis of the neuroendocrine system. It controls the secretion of pituitary hormones, including gonadotropins, adrenocorticotropic hormone, thyroid-stimulating hormone, growth hormone, and prolactin.

One of the most important hormones for patients undergoing the pathophysiology of brain death is the synthesis of arginine vasopressin, which is sent through the axon to the posterior pituitary and released into circulation. Vasopressin maintains the homeostasis of plasma osmotic pressure. When this hormone becomes insufficient, diabetes insipidus (DI) follows. While DI is frequently seen in patients with brain death who continue to receive ventilator support, Nair-Collins's group demonstrated that up to about half of the reported cases showed detectable vasopressin blood level, consistent with at least partially functioning hypothalamus [27]. Moreover, while quantification is difficult, reported cases of long-term somatic support after the diagnosis of brain death demonstrated puberty, menstruation, body growth, and temperature regulation, all of which would have been impossible without at least partially functioning hypothalamus and the pituitary gland.

3.2 Three options for revision

Given the possible survival of the hypothalamus after the diagnosis of brain death, there are roughly three options to address this problem. First, the test for the hypothalamic function is included in the revised UDDA to maintain the language of "all functions of the entire brain." For example, the law will read, "... including the brainstem and hypothalamus." The second option is to abandon the concept of "all functions of the entire brain" and to narrow the anatomical area to the brain stem, leaving off the cerebrum, including the hypothalamus, and the cerebellum without direct evaluation. This definition has been adopted in the code of practice for the diagnosis of death in the United Kingdom (UK) and is often called "irreversible apneic unresponsiveness," an apt syndromic name. The third option is to keep the status quo, acknowledging that the hypothalamic function may remain in some cases. It is also possible to keep the current wording except for adding, "... excluding the hypothalamus."

The proposed revision seems to combine the second and third options above [5]. The proposal keeps the current "all functions of the entire brain" but adds "leading to unresponsive coma with loss of capacity for consciousness, brainstem areflexia and the inability to breathe spontaneously." This version works in both ways: It is still about "all functions of the entire brain," but the focus is only apneic unresponsiveness. It ignores the hypothalamus, but if it is challenged about its preservation, one could contend that "the focus is only the brain stem and apnea, not hormones." At the same time, if it is challenged that this revision narrows brain death from the whole brain criteria to the brain stem criteria, it tries to escape the challenge by saying that the revision still keeps the language of "all functions of the entire brain." They also propose a backup option to explicitly exclude "hormonal function" while keeping the whole brain language.

The first option to include the hypothalamus in "all functions of the entire brain" may not be seriously considered, probably because such a change requires the assessment of the hypothalamic function to be added to the protocol of brain death diagnosis. Such an addition would be a new challenge because the irreversible cessation of the hypothalamic function is probably more difficult to establish promptly than other brain functions, and further research is likely necessary.

3.3 Ethical analysis of the brain region to be evaluated

If the proposed revision that does not mention the hypothalamus but adds the language of apneic unresponsive coma were adopted, it would certainly face above mentioned challenges. The replies would be evasive at best and could be outright contradictory in that "all functions of the entire brain" is subtly narrowed to exclude the hypothalamic hormonal function and focus only on the brain stem and apnea. This version would not escape the criticism of an *ad hoc* makeshift revision only to smother the inconvenient fact.[4]

Nevertheless, as mentioned earlier, "brain stem death" has been adopted in the UK all along [30]. This definition narrows down the brain region required to cease functioning irreversibly to the brain stem. One advantage of brain stem death is that the US definition becomes streamlined with the UK definition, foreshadowing the worldwide standardization of diagnosing brain death. Historically, there was a debate across the Atlantic in the 1970s and early 80s whether the brain stem criteria in the UK are equivalent to the whole brain criteria in the US. The difference between these two criteria appeared very significant, and some US physicians argued that the UK criteria would misclassify those who might recover later. There were anecdotal cases from the US where those diagnosed as brain death by the UK criteria were not quite brain dead, though these cases were later disputed [31].

In the end, however, this difference is, technically speaking, not so significant. First, these definitions only refer to the function, not the pathology of the brain. Brain stem death does not mean the pathology is limited to the brain stem. It only means that the evaluation is limited to the loss of brain stem functions, deep unresponsiveness, and positive apnea test. Second, the rest of the brain is inferred to have ceased to function based on the depth of coma, confirmation of severe enough lesions inside the skull by imaging tests, and exclusion of other miscellaneous conditions that mimic brain death. Historically, this is how the UK criteria evaluated the cerebrum, albeit indirectly, without ancillary tests such as EEG. In contrast, the US criteria for many years used ancillary tests, particularly EEG and brain blood flow tests, to ensure

[4] Karl Popper, one of the most influential philosophers of science, considers an *ad hoc* theory repair in the face of falsifying evidence is a mark of pseudoscience [29].

there is no electrical or perfusion activity in the cerebrum. However, in recent years, particularly after the revision of the American Academy of Neurology (AAN) guidelines in 2010, which discouraged ancillary testing except when a clinical examination is incomplete, the US guidelines are very similar to that of the UK.

The most important ethical question is whether the actual practice is what the UDDA stipulates. If the language of "all functions of the entire brain" is kept unchanged, yet in practice, the protocol leaves out the hypothalamus, it is a downright contradiction. For this reason, it is also possible to adopt a narrower version of the brain stem death and abandon "all functions of the entire brain." Conceptually speaking, it is impossible for all brain regions at once to stop functioning at the time of diagnosis. Additional areas of functional survival can be discovered in some cases of brain death. Whether this fact is acceptable is a matter of value judgment and something physicians alone cannot and should not decide. It should be evaluated by those involved in the decision through informed consent and eventually by the informed public. Such uncertainty and inevitable imperfection of the diagnosis are more of the reason that informed consent and conscientious exemption are indispensable in diagnosing brain death.

4. Codification of the guidelines published by the AAN and affiliated organizations as the sole authority of the "accepted medical standards"

The proposed revision suggests codifying the current guidelines for brain death diagnosis published by the AAN and affiliated professional organizations as the sole standards. These guidelines would replace the "accepted medical standards" in the current UDDA. While most neurologists follow the AAN guidelines of 1995 [32] and its updated 2010 version [33], some specialists other than neurologists and particularly older practitioners still use the predecessor of the AAN guidelines, the Harvard criteria of 1968 [3].

The major differences between the Harvard Criteria and the AAN Guidelines are twofold: The former strongly recommends confirmatory EEG, which should be flat, and a repeat examination in 24 hours is required. When the UDDA was issued in 1981, medical consultants of the President's Committee published their guidelines based on the UDDA in JAMA 1981 [34]. It was almost identical to the Harvard criteria, except that the observation period was shortened from 24 to 12 hours, except for anoxic brain damage. For example, one of the most authoritative textbooks of neurology, *Principles of Neurology* by Adams and Victor [35], gives the following instruction on the diagnosis of brain death in 1985, 4 years after the UDDA was released:

> *The EEG is a valuable indicator of cerebral death and most institutions require proof of electrocerebral silence (ECS), also called a flat or isoelectric EEG ... When examination has disclosed that all brain functions are absent, it should be repeated in 6 h, to confirm that the state is irreversible (p. 258).*

The first version of AAN Guidelines 1995 still recommended a repeat clinical evaluation 6 hours later, but it is now "optional." Confirmatory tests are "not mandatory but desirable," though EEG was no longer the first choice, replaced by cerebral angiography [32].

In the update of 2010, a repeat examination is no longer recommended, and an ancillary test is not required except when the clinical examination is incomplete for various reasons [33]. This progressive minimization of the protocol bewilders those who have practiced neurology for decades. The only reason to justify this change is the assertion that there has been no case of diagnostic error (or classifying patients who are not dead as dead). As many critiques have already pointed out [36], and even the President's Council recognized [37], the current practice of diagnosing brain death is a self-fulfilling prophesy: The patient is dead because we diagnosed so. There is no independent proof that such a diagnosis is not false positive because the evidence is all erased by promptly disposing of the body or subjecting it to organ procurement. As mentioned in 2.3, anecdotal cases of diagnostic errors have been reported [19, 20]. Moreover, the AAN's main journal, *Neurology*, reported many reports of non-compliance to their guidelines [16–18].

Why has this ethical problem of the AAN guidelines persisted? The reason is that the guidelines were not created in a moral vacuum. It cannot remove itself from underlying professional interests: efficiency and ease of use. As mentioned in 2.4.3, the proponents of the AAN guidelines are eager to save resources by promptly disposing of any patients who might have brain death. The history of the brain death guidelines shows this priority of efficiency: The number of physicians was reduced from two to one, the number of examinations was reduced from two to one, and the use of ancillary tests was minimized from strongly recommended to none unless necessary. The only justification is always the same: no reported case of diagnostic error, even when there is no way of identifying diagnostic error.

However, as any physicians who have had the most basic education of the sensitivity and specificity of diagnostic tests know, if the specificity of a test is crucial, such as classifying the patient dead as opposed to alive, the test should have the highest specificity even at the cost of sensitivity. In other words, even if we may miss a case that is truly brain dead as still alive, we want to and must be positive not to misclassify a single case that is still alive as brain dead. A simple calculation of the specificity of repeat testing shows that the overall specificity of repeated testing is always greater than singular testing. If one wants to make sure to achieve the highest specificity, even if we do not know the value of specificity itself, repeating the test always increases the specificity and thus safety.[5]

There is always a risk in legally authorizing one organization or a vested interest group as the sole authority of critically important medical practice. It is, of course, natural and understandable to maximize their vested interest, but there should be checks and balances against the inherent conflict of interest. At a minimum, such guidelines require close oversight by entirely independent ethicists and laypeople who have not participated in any practice of the legal, medical, or ethical aspect of diagnosing brain death. Such an oversight organization is critically important to judge whether the protocol is ethically acceptable given the nature of this diagnostic test, which defies formal evaluation for its safety, specificity, and sensitivity required for any other medical tests.

[5] Suppose Sp1 is the specificity of the first test, Sp2 is that of the second test, and Sp1&2 is the cumulative specificity of repeated test 1 and test 2 (we assume that Sp1 and Sp2 are different because the first and second brain death evaluation has different specificities due to rapidly changing condition of those patients). $Sp1\&2 = 1 - [(1-Sp1) * (1-Sp2)] = Sp1 + Sp2 - Sp1*Sp2$. This value is always greater than Sp1 or Sp2 alone; thus, the specificity of repeated testing (Sp1&2) is always greater than singular testing (Sp1 or Sp2). It is also the rationale to increase the specificity of a negative COVID-19 home test by repeating it in 48 hours.

5. Insights into the ethical controversies behind the revision of the UDDA

5.1 Value or science

Several insights from this brief review can be extracted. The first insight is that the fundamental problem of the "science" behind the diagnosis of brain death is that it is "unscientific." The diagnosis of brain death is indeed based on a large body of accumulated scientific knowledge regarding severe and devastating brain damage. That is not an issue. The issue is that the science of brain death confuses itself, whether intentionally or unintentionally, with a fundamental value judgment of what constitutes life and death. Humanity has many millennia of experiences and moral intuition to classify who is alive and dead. No doctors or scientists are required to classify these two distinct conditions. It has been done without any medical knowledge throughout the history of humanity. The alleged science of brain death has imposed its value in the name and the "clothing" of science to override this fundamental moral intuition.

It is sometimes pointed out that the debate over brain death parallels the debate over abortion. Of course, there is a morally relevant difference between the two. In abortion, the values of two lives (mother vs. fetus) are involved, whereas, in brain death, it is the value of the life of one brain-damaged person. However, an important moral feature is common in both abortion and brain death. It is primarily a value decision, not a medical or scientific decision. No amount of scientific and medical argument can overturn the underlying value judgment. Abortion seems to have already been treated under this assumption, yet the ethical debate of brain death has not reached this maturity. We are still under the illusion that, somehow, the science of brain death can tell that it is a person's death. Under this illusion, those who do not accept brain death are considered "uneducated, unscientific"; therefore, their voices can be silenced by the legal and medical authorities. The proposal under review by the ULA suggests that the proponents of this revision want to enforce that brain death is primarily a medical and legal decision, and the value judgment of the patients and families is pushed behind. Of course, that does not mean that personal values can define human death any way we want. We already have an excellent universal definition of death: circulatory death. Most people do not want to propose any further complex definition of death; most just want to die with a default definition, and indeed most do.

5.2 Brain death as a critically important and necessary instrument of medicine

What is the actual value of diagnosing brain death, then? Why must we diagnose brain death as soon as it is suspected in a patient with a devastating brain injury? The insight given from this review is that we need to come to this fundamental question. The answer is a logical consequence of what we have been doing over the past several decades: It is almost entirely to conserve healthcare resources and procure vital organs for transplantation. Diagnosing brain death is now an indispensable *tool* for these important utilitarian goals. Besides, there is nothing inherently and morally wrong in pursuing these goals *per se*. What is morally wrong with the proponents of the current proposal of denying consent and neglecting the specificity of the brain death testing is to disguise this practice as morally equivalent to diagnosing traditional circulatory death by making the practice *appear* "symmetrical" between brain death and circulatory death. Their naive logic is that because we do not do this for circulatory death, we should not do this for brain death. Because of this superficial disguise by arranging the same practice for circulatory death and brain death, many inconsistencies came out through legal cases and falsifying clinical cases. Instead of further enforcing this false narrative through legislation, it is necessary to come down to the actual goals of this medical practice: an ethical disposition of cases with devastating brain injury with dismal prognoses and heart-beating organ donations.

5.3 Pragmatic solutions to the current difficulties of brain death practice through informed consent

The above two insights, brain death as a value judgment and brain death as a crucial utilitarian instrument, suggest that informed consent before diagnosing brain death can solve most difficulties that the current effort to revise the UDDA addresses [38]. It is a *voluntary* contribution to the utilitarian goals through the consenting process. In other words, consenting patients are volunteering to be heart-beating organ donors through the diagnosis of brain death due to an extremely poor prognosis, whether or not they believe that brain death is equivalent to circulatory death for them.

5.3.1 Consent can subsume religious and conscientious exemption before the diagnosis

The first advantage of consent is that, as discussed in detail in 2.5, it takes place immediately before the procedure is prepared. The process of informed consent is a bidirectional information exchange, and what is discussed is entirely specific to what has happened to the patient here and now, as opposed to a hypothetical and abstract consideration about something that may not happen at all. Whether the exemption is religious, cultural, conscientious, or technical, the answer is the same: They are all given a chance to say "no" at the moment of the final pathway. Since the diagnosis of brain death never happens if the consent is declined, those patients who want to claim exemptions can have their end-of-life care most appropriate to their cultural and personal values instead of being labeled as "brain dead" after a diagnosis as Jahi McMath was.

5.3.2 Consent can facilitate organ donation of consented heart-beating donors

Informed consent can also facilitate heart-beating organ donation. For those donors, it is crucially important to perform the diagnostic protocol of brain death promptly to meet their wishes to donate fresh organs for successful transplantation. At the same time, diagnosing brain death has no value for non-organ donors, whether by preference or for medical reasons. For them, it is entirely unnecessary. The current practice of nondiscriminatory brain death testing wastes precious medical resources. Those cases should eventually be transitioned to palliative comfort care to die peacefully from cardiac arrest instead of inhumane, unnecessary brain death testing followed by unilaterally removing life support and forcing the heart to stop. Additionally, those who might be organ donors but are undecided about the diagnosis of brain death might be good candidates for non-heart-beating donation, and this can be offered along with the option for palliative care.

5.3.3 Consent can cover other issues being considered in this revision

Consent is a powerful tool for information exchange. If the conference is appropriately held, the topic of brain region can be briefly discussed. Whether the whole brain formulation or the brain stem formulation is adopted, it is impossible to ensure that all the brain tissue is dead at diagnosis. The family and surrogate should have a good understanding that the diagnosis of brain death is only through "sampling" the functions of the brain stem to infer the death of the entire brain. Whether the hypothalamus is included or not, some part of the brain might inevitably remain functioning, and the decision-makers should be aware of this prior to consent. It is an inherent risk that a consented patient needs to accept. The consenting conference could also cover the problem of the AAN protocol. While we are using this protocol, the medical team could repeat the test in 6–24 hours to ensure the reproducibility and specificity of the result by simply calculating the specificity of the test, even if the AAN protocol does not require it. Conscientious practitioners can meet the desire of the family if they want. As long as the family and prospective patients in public understand the risk involved in diagnosing brain death, the consenting process can safeguard against the excessive and overzealous application of brain death diagnosis.

6. The final thoughts and conclusion

Over the past 40-plus years, the UDDA has succeeded in one sense but failed in another. It is a success in enabling heart-beating organ donation that saved countless lives. At the same time, it created persistent moral and philosophical dissensions due to the unsettled epistemic and metaphysical nature of brain death. To overcome persistent disagreements, the proponents of the current practice made every effort to convince the public that brain death is not just a state of the brain but death that is no different from the irreversible stoppage of the heart and respiration. That is proven to be a failure. The underlying metaphysical and epistemic differences between brain death and circulatory death are unmistakably conspicuous to the families witnessing every detail of the loved one being diagnosed as brain dead. No amount of science can convince those families that the warm and perspiring body with a beating heart is medically the same as a cold and rigid corpse that died of circulatory death. It is those families who persisted in the deeply-held intuition of human life, those who questioned the fundamental discrepancy and raised voices and brought the case to the judicial system, and it is such families that shook up the established system of brain death backed by the UDDA.

There are limited options if our society wishes to continue heart-beating organ donation from brain-dead donors. Making *ad hoc* adjustments, such as excluding hypothalamic function while precluding the patient and family from opting out of the definition and practice of brain death by eliminating consent, is an option pursued by the proponents of the current practice. As we reviewed, there is a better way to solve all disagreements: allowing the personal choice of death determination through consent and exemption. With this simple and well-established ethical practice, there will be no need for the ethically objectionable practice of imposing the diagnosis of brain death against the wishes of families and surrogates. At the same time, willing patients and families, particularly consenting organ donors, have full access to the diagnosis of brain death followed by organ donation. So long as all risks and imperfections of the diagnosis are accepted through the consenting process, there is nothing inherently and morally objectionable to continuing the current definition and the practice of diagnosing brain death as a *tool* to facilitate heart-beating organ donation without violating the dead-donor rule. On the other hand, precluding personal choice and imposing legal restrictions to consent would further erode public trust. Regardless of the outcome of the revision, these ethical debates will and should continue beyond the current revision, probably at state levels.

Author details

Osamu Muramoto
Center for Ethics in Health Care, Oregon Health and Science University,
Portland, OR, USA

*Address all correspondence to: muramoto@ohsu.edu

References

[1] Uniform Law Commission [Internet]. Available from: https://www.uniformlaws.org/ [Accessed: May 25, 2023]

[2] Burkle CM, Pope TM. Brain death: Legal obligations and the courts. Seminars in Neurology. 2015;**35**:174-179

[3] A definition of irreversible coma. Report of the ad hoc Committee of the Harvard Medical School to examine the definition of brain death. Journal of the American Medical Association. 1968;**205**(6):337-340

[4] Truog RD, Berlinger N, Zacharias RL, Solomon MZ. Brain death at fifty: Exploring consensus, controversy, and contexts. The Hastings Center Report. 2018;**48**(Suppl 4):S2-S5

[5] Lewis A, Bonnie RJ, Pope T, et al. Determination of death by neurologic criteria in the United States: The case for revising the uniform determination of death act. The Journal of Law, Medicine & Ethics. 2019;**47**(4_suppl):9-24

[6] Veatch RM, Ross LF. Defining Death: The Case for Choice. Washington: Georgetown University Press; 2016

[7] Bagheri A. Individual choice in the definition of death. Journal of Medical Ethics. 2007;**33**(3):146-149

[8] New Jersey Revised Statutes § 26:6A-4, 5

[9] New York Codes, Rules and Regulations § 400.16(c)-(e)

[10] California Code, Health and Safety Code § 1254.4

[11] Illinois Statute 210 ILCS. § 85/6.24

[12] Morison RS. Death: Process or event? Science. 1971;**173**(3998):694-698

[13] Lewis A, Pope TM. Physician power to declare death by neurologic criteria threatened. Neurocritical Care. 2017;**26**(3):446-449

[14] Nevada Revised Statute § 451.008

[15] Muramoto O. Informed consent for the diagnosis of brain death: A conceptual argument. Philosophy, Ethics, and Humanities in Medicine. 2016;**11**(1):8

[16] Greer DM, Varelas PN, Haque S, Wijdicks EF. Variability of brain death determination guidelines in leading US neurologic institutions. Neurology. 2008;**70**:284-289

[17] Bartscher JF, Varelas PN. Determining brain death—no room for error. Virtual Mentor. 2010;**12**:879-884

[18] Shappell CN, Frank JI, Husari K, Sanchez M, Goldenberg F, Ardelt A. Practice variability in brain death determination: A call to action. Neurology. 2013;**81**:2009-2014

[19] Shewmon DA. False-positive diagnosis of brain death following the pediatric guidelines: Case report and discussion. Journal of Child Neurology. 2017;**32**(14):1104-1117

[20] Shewmon DA. Statement in support of revising the uniform determination of death act and in opposition to a proposed revision [published online ahead of print, 2021 May 14]. Journal of Medicine and Philosophy. 2021:jhab014. DOI: 10.1093/jmp/jhab014

[21] Joffe AR, Anton NR, Duff JP. The apnea test: Rationale, confounders, and

criticism. Journal of Child Neurology. 2010;**25**(11):1435-1443

[22] Lewis A, Bonnie RJ, Pope T. Is there a right to delay determination of death by neurologic criteria? JAMA Neurology. 2020;**77**(11):1347-1348

[23] Shewmon DA, Salamon N. The extraordinary case of Jahi McMath. Perspectives in Biology and Medicine. 2021;**64**(4):457-478

[24] Yadav KN, Gabler NB, Cooney E, et al. Approximately one in three US adults completes any type of advance directive for end-of-life care. Health Affairs (Millwood). 2017;**36**(7):1244-1251

[25] Shah SK, Kasper K, Miller FG. A narrative review of the empirical evidence on public attitudes on brain death and vital organ transplantation: The need for better data to inform policy. Journal of Medical Ethics. 2015;**41**(4):291-296

[26] Kondziella D, Stevens RD. Classifying disorders of consciousness: Past, present, and future. Seminars in Neurology. 2022;**42**(3):239-248

[27] Nair-Collins M, Northrup J, Olcese J. Hypothalamic-pituitary function in brain death: A review. Journal of Intensive Care Medicine. 2016;**31**(1):41-50

[28] Nair-Collins M, Joffe AR. Frequent preservation of neurologic function in brain death and brainstem death entails false-positive misdiagnosis and cerebral perfusion [published online ahead of print, 2021 Sep 29]. AJOB Neuroscience. 2021:1-14

[29] Popper KR. Conjectures and Refutations; the Growth of Scientific Knowledge. New York: Basic Books; 1962

[30] The Academy of Medical Royal Colleges. A Code of Practice for the Diagnosis and Confirmation of Death. A report of the Academy of Medical Royal Colleges; 2008. Available from https://www.aomrc.org.uk/wp-content/uploads/2016/04/Code_Practice_Confirmation_Diagnosis_Death_1008-4.pdf

[31] Wijdicks EF. The transatlantic divide over brain death determination and the debate. Brain. 2012;**135**(Pt 4):1321-1331

[32] Practice parameters for determining brain death in adults (summary statement). The quality standards Subcommittee of the American Academy of neurology. Neurology. 1995;**45**(5):1012-1014

[33] Wijdicks EF, Varelas PN, Gronseth GS, Greer DM, American Academy of Neurology. Evidence-based guideline update: Determining brain death in adults: Report of the quality standards Subcommittee of the American Academy of neurology. Neurology. 2010;**74**(23):1911-1918

[34] Guidelines for the determination of death. Report of the medical consultants on the diagnosis of death to the President's Commission for the Study of ethical problems in medicine and biomedical and behavioral research. Journal of the American Medical Association. 1981;**246**(19):2184-2186

[35] Adams RD, Victor M. Principles of Neurology. 3rd ed. New York: McGraw Hill Book; 1985

[36] Truog RD, Robinson WM. Role of brain death and the dead-donor rule in the ethics of organ transplantation. Critical Care Medicine. 2003;**31**(9):2391-2396

[37] President's Council on Bioethics. Controversies in the Determination of

Death. Washington, DC: President's Council on Bioethics; 2008

[38] Muramoto O. Is informed consent required for the diagnosis of brain death regardless of consent for organ donation? [published online ahead of print, 2020 Jun 5]. Journal of Medical Ethics. 2020;**47**(12):e5

Chapter 6

Postmortem Interval Ocular Indicators

Sandra Vianney Ramírez Ojeda and Cesar Hernandez Mier

Abstract

Postmortem interval, the time elapsed since the death of a body, is critical in determining the investigations of unwitnessed deaths. Therefore, it is a fundamental variable that has been investigated for numerous years. The eye is one of the readiest organs to assess; thus, it becomes very convenient when analyzing a corpse at a crime scene. Several cadaveric phenomena have been described in the eyes, which can be observed in different structures such as the cornea, sclera, iris, lens, vitreous body, retina, and intraocular pressure. These phenomena can, directly and indirectly, contribute to determining the postmortem interval, and so have other quantitative and reproducible elements that collaborate in investigating deaths without witnesses, including deaths in hospitals or at home, and with this to be able to resolve trials. Consequently, in the next chapter, we will review the elements necessary to determine postmortem interval, considering cadaveric phenomena occurring at an ocular level.

Keywords: post-mortem interval, ocular indicators, cadaveric phenomena, ocular changes, after death

1. Introduction

The emergence of forensic sciences is born out of the law's necessity of answering questions, which, although they originate within the law, have found a basis in other sciences. Therefore, throughout history, the law has incorporated sciences that have contributed to answering those questions that the law raises to solve the problems it addresses. Such a set of sciences is known as the forensic sciences.

Likewise, it is essential to highlight that a large number of questions for which the law demands an answer have a basis in time; that is, they are questions that seek to know elements associated with time, for example, the date of a laceration, the age of an individual, the time it takes for lacerations to heal, and even the date of death.

These types of questions are not new. We can say that, since the dawn of law, humans have attempted to solve one of the crucial questions associated with time: when did a given person lose their life? We have tried to implement procedures such as qualitatively describing cadaveric phenomena, determining metabolites, and other more sophisticated methods.

However, the evolution of science and so-called evidence-based medicine has led to questioning many of these procedures that were considered valid until a few years ago. Therefore, we have conducted actions that allow quantitative parameters with

 IntechOpen

narrow and known margin errors to determine postmortem interval. For this reason, this chapter reviews the methods for estimating the postmortem interval from ocular parameters.

2. Postmortem interval

Indeed, one of the main objectives during the practice of a necropsy is determining the moment in which a person dies, understood as the period that elapses from the moment a person loses his life to the moment the body is found, or an expert practices an intervention. Consequently, its importance is such that, in some cases, it could determine the responsibility, or lack thereof, of a person in the death of an individual.

The commonly used term in medical forensics is estimated postmortem interval (PMI); however, postmortem window is the term of choice in some places. Its usefulness lies not only in estimating how long a body has been dead but in distinguishing antemortem from postmortem trauma. Thus, in most homicide cases or unwitnessed death investigations (including in-hospital deaths), it is a crucial step since it is essential to include and exclude suspects. Therefore, it remains one of the most critical, and challenging to quantify and establish, variables despite widely conducted research [1, 2].

3. Cadaveric phenomena

Techniques currently used to estimate PMI are very diverse. Most have focused on the qualitative analysis of cadaveric phenomena (**Table 1**), which we can define as traces left by death. Their study contributes to estimating PMI. Among the critical phenomena classified as abiotic are cadaveric lividity [4], often described as one of the first signs of death; cadaveric rigidity or rigor mortis [5]; thermal exchange with the environment; and dehydration process. The latter is caused by the evaporation of body fluids and is observed mainly in body weight, skin, mucous membranes, and at an ocular level [6, 7].

1. Methods Based on Temperature Measurement
2. Other Methods
a. Supravitality Phenomena
i. Ocular Changes
ii. Mechanical Excitability
iii. Electric Excitability
b. Changes in Muscles and Tissue
i. Cadaveric Rigidity
ii. Hypostasis
c. Assessment of Gastric Content
d. Tanathochemical Methods

Table 1.
Classification of methods of estimating early postmortem interval [3].

It is precisely the cadaveric phenomenon (CF) of dehydration, specifically the process of dehydration at an ocular level, that we will be addressing in this work, which is why it is essential to analyze some basic principles of ocular anatomy.

4. Ocular anatomy

Although critical elements can be collected from the examination of the eyes of a cadaver, the latter are not routinely subjected to in-depth analysis since ocular pathology is an important challenge for non-specialist physicians in the area. So, before delving into ocular cadaveric phenomena, it is of the essence to acquire basic ocular anatomy knowledge and the nomenclature used by ophthalmologists to describe injuries, pathologies, and ocular phenomena. This knowledge will improve doctor-examiner communications. For a better anatomical description of the eyeball and its annexes, we will describe it from the outside along an axial plane (**Figure 1**).

- *Eyelids:* They are the outermost and protective structure of the eyeball, they are composed of the thinnest skin of the human body, the orbicularis oculi muscle in its preseptal and pretarsal portion, and the tarsus (a cartilaginous structure that contains the glands of meibomian), in the upper eyelid is the levator muscle of the eyelid, which as its name suggests, helps to raise the eyelid and the eyelid opening [9, 10].

- *Orbit:* It is a rigid pear-shaped cavity that protects the structures of the eyeball and comprises four bone walls: superior, inferior, lateral, and medial walls [9].

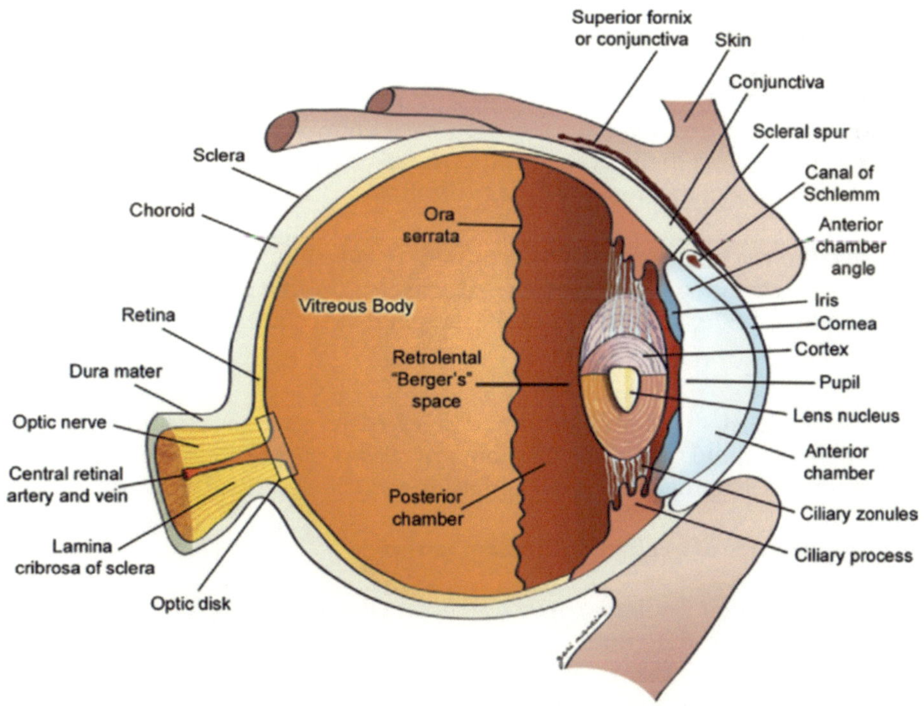

Figure 1.
Diagrammatic representation of the gross anatomy of the globe [8].

- *Conjunctiva:* A transparent mucous membrane that covers the inner surface of the eyelids and the anterior surface of the eyeball, ends at the corneoscleral limbus, and has abundant vascularization from the anterior and palpebral ciliary arteries. Its function is mainly protective, intervening in passive and active immunity [9, 10].

- *Cornea*: It is a complex and transparent structure composed of five layers (from anterior to posterior): epithelium, Bowman's layer (a membrane that limits and protects internal tissues), stroma, Descemet's membrane, and endothelium. In addition to fulfilling a protective mission, it is responsible for three-fourths of the eye's optical power. It lacks blood vessels, but it is the body tissue with the highest nerve density. Moreover, it nourishes itself through the aqueous humor in the anterior chamber. Its thickness averages 500 microns, but it is a strong and stable fabric [9].

- *Anterior chamber*: The space between the iris and the cornea contains aqueous humor, a transparent liquid produced by the ciliary processes that nourish the cornea [9, 10].

- *Iris:* It constitutes a muscular membranous tissue that functions as a diaphragm inside the eye. The central opening, the pupil, can vary its diameter: miosis (constriction) occurs to reduce light entry; and mydriasis, to increase light entry.

- *Sclera:* The scleral stroma is composed of collagen bundles of various sizes and shapes that are not oriented uniformly with the cornea, so it is not transparent but white; the inner layer of the sclera fuses with the uvea. It also provides rigidity and support to the eyeball [9, 10].

- *Vitreous:* It is a transparent extracellular gel formed by collagen, soluble proteins, hyaluronic acid, and water. Its total volume is approximately 4 mL, it provides structural support to the eyeball and at the same time, it is a transparent and optically uniform medium for light to reach the retina.

- *Retina:* It is the inner layer of the eye that is responsible for transmitting nervous and visual stimuli to the optic nerve, it also contains the macula, a structure of the posterior pole, located within the temporal vascular arcades and provides the central vision of the eye [10].

At an ocular level, different indicators can help determine the circumstances or events the corpse could have gone through, pre- and post-mortem. These can occur in all the structures forming the eyeball and its previously described annexes.

4.1 The importance of evaluating ocular trauma

Postmortem ocular findings can be instrumental in estimating postmortem interval. We must first determine and assess the integrity of ocular structures and their annexes in a given corpse. Since such trauma is a frequent occurrence in physical aggressions, work incidents, and traffic accidents—the leading causes of unwitnessed deaths—conducting an initial assessment to decide whether or not the integrity of the eyeball will help determine the postmortem interval.

Injuries to be assessed are listed according to the affected anatomical area:

- *Eyelids:* Possible injuries in the eyelids include lacerations (continuity solution) **Figure 2A**, palpebral ecchymosis, and palpebral edema. If any of these three is present, a complete evaluation will be necessary to rule out rupture or laceration to the eyeball [11].

- *Cornea:* It will be necessary to open the eyelids to assess the integrity of the cornea and determine if there are abrasions, corneal erosions, or corneal opacity (which may be related to chemical burns), or corneal foreign bodies (**Figure 2B**). This assessment is essential because it can completely change the cadaveric phenomena after death; pathologies may cause opacity before death, such as absolute glaucoma, corneal hydrops, corneal transplant rejection, corneal ulcers, or scars. In addition, when there are full-thickness corneal injuries, intraocular pressure can decrease significantly, and on the contrary, when there is hyphema or traumatic uveitis, (**Figure 2C–D**) intraocular pressure might increase. In such situations, we shall not consider the pressure measurement as a determining factor of postmortem interval [10].

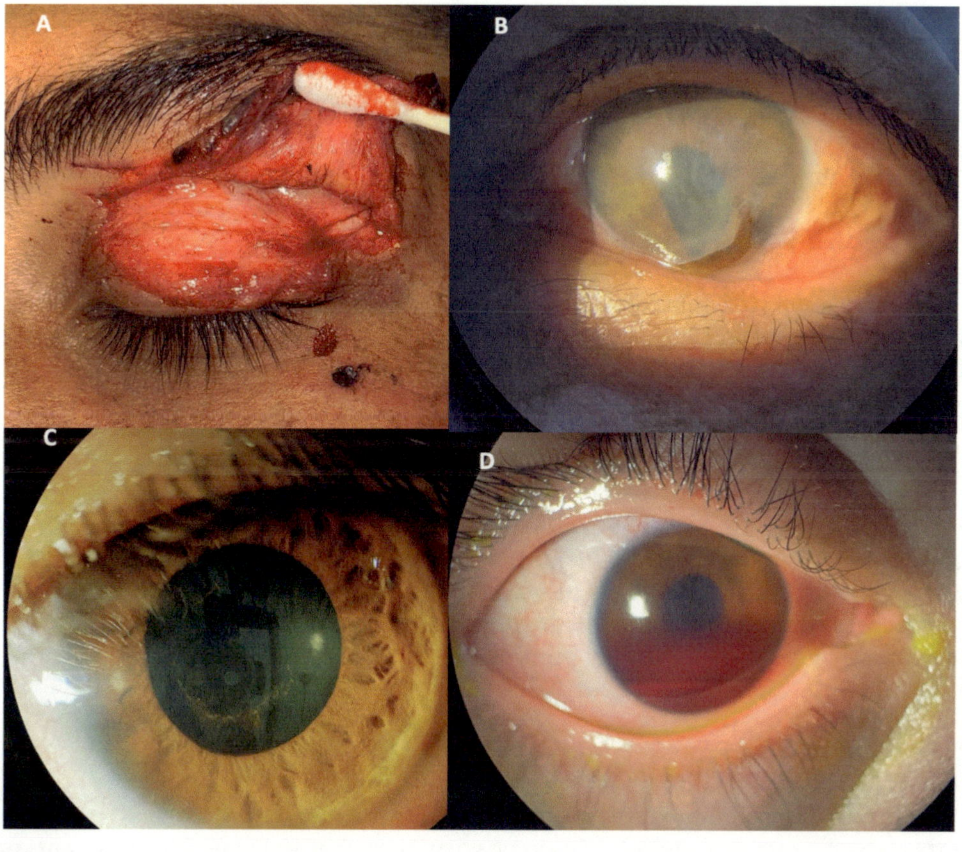

Figure 2.
Ocular traumatisms that can modify ocular cadaveric phenomena. A.- Eyelid laceration. B. Full-thickness corneal laceration with iris protrusion. C.- Vossius ring secondary to swelling in anterior chamber (traumatic uveitis) D.- Hyphema (blood in anterior chamber).

- *Conjunctiva*: As previously described, this is a significantly irrigated layer. In traumatic situations, subconjunctival hemorrhages (hyposphagma) or hemorrhagic chemosis are infrequent; in the case of the latter, it must rule out rupture of the eyeball.

- *Anterior chamber:* A complete evaluation of the iris, beginning with the pupils, can give significant clues. Spastic miosis is frequently associated with ocular trauma and is generally transient. In contrast, mydriasis may be associated with rupture of the pupillary sphincter or traumatic uveitis, which can modify intraocular pressure and the characteristics of the ocular postmortem process. Hyphema (blood deposited in the anterior chamber) can also cause increased intraocular pressure and modify this parameter as a postmortem indicator.

- *Lens:* Traumatic cataract formation following direct trauma to the eyeball can cause complete opacification of the lens.

- *Vitreous:* At the vitreous level, it will be necessary to assess its transparency because there could be a hemorrhage in the vitreous cavity after a trauma (hemovitreous) which would prevent us from assessing the retina and retinal cadaveric phenomena.

- *Retina*: Ocular trauma—from retinal contusion, retinal dialysis, and retinal detachment to choroidal detachment—may seem unclear at first sight. The latter can change the external assessment of the eyeball, causing ocular hypotonia.

- *Orbit:* At the orbital level, ethmoid and orbital floor fractures are common in ocular trauma and are usually associated with signs related to other ocular structures [11].

The above shows that before considering cadaveric phenomena at the ocular level, we must rule out the existence of ocular trauma since this will substantially modify the interpretation of the ocular cadaveric phenomenon.

5. Ocular cadaveric phenomena

The determination of postmortem interval is a crucial parameter in medicolegal cases and unwitnessed deaths. One of the most convenient anatomical sites in forensic investigations is the eyes because it is an easily accessible area for analysis. Therefore, a complete initial assessment of the eyeball and its annexes will have to be exhaustive so that the eyes can provide the necessary information regarding the time of death.

5.1 Loss of corneal transparency or corneal opacity

As previously mentioned, the corneal structure is a translucent tissue. However, as the date of death evolves, it begins to opacify, caused by the deposit of remnants of softened and detached corneal epithelium. This phenomenon is relatively early. Still, it is the beginning of a sequence of events like those described by Nori in 2018, which we can see in **Table 2** [12, 13].

Hours post-mortem	Main findings at OCT analysis
<2	Decrease in corneal thickness
	Increase in epithelial reflectivity
2–6	Increase in thickness of corneal stroma
	Increase in endothelial reflectivity
	Visible differentiation in reflectivity between the anterior and posterior stromal segments
6–12	Corneal swelling
	Delamination of the stroma
12–24	Decrease in depth of anterior chamber
	Disappearance of the epithelium
	Formation of hypo-reflective areas
24–48	Decrease in depth of anterior chamber
	Decrease in corneal curvature
	Disappearance of the epithelium
48–72	Iris and cornea tended to collapse
	Posterior stroma tended to vacuolise
	Formation of subepithelial bubbles
	Formation of hyper-reflective dots (debris) in the aqueous humor

Table 2.
Main findings in the cornea according to the postmortem hours described by Nioi et al. [12].

The association between the loss of corneal transparency with the time elapsed since death was established in 1965 by Aoki et al., who reported that the cornea remained transparent for 8 to 12 postmortem hours. However, signs of opacity became evident in 15% of cases between 12 and 18 postmortem hours, 25% of cases between 18 and 24 postmortem hours, and 75% of cases between 24 and 36 postmortem hours [14]. In 1970, Wroblewski and Ellis reported that minimal corneal opacity was visible at two postmortem hours in 74% of cases, thus concluding that the total absence of this phenomenon indicates that death occurred within the two previous hours [15].

We must analyze this information critically must be analyzed while highlighting its limitations. On the one hand, corneal opacity is a qualitative variable at this time, so it is subject to the observer's appreciation and the conditions in which the observation was conducted. In turn, it may be affected depending if the eyes were kept closed or open after death. Weather variations affect it directly; even humidity and extreme heat can generate early corneal opacity.

5.2 Changes in pupil diameter

After death, the photomotor reflex (pupillary constriction produced by light) cannot be stimulated, so pupils usually present median mydriasis. Pharmacological agents such as acetylcholine and tropicamide do not affect this phenomenon; therefore, we should consider using changes in pupil size to estimate the postmortem interval with great caution; we must remember that, if there was ocular trauma, the rupture in the iris sphincter could change this assessment [16].

6. Apparition of scleral spots

We may describe it as a black spot with poorly defined contours that appears on the outer side of the eyeball, emerging posteriorly. The spot tends to spread transversely and is not an absolute constant; it is caused by desiccation of the sclera, which produces its thinning, allowing the observation of the uveal tissue (choroid) [17]. As similarly referred to in corneal opacity, this is a qualitative variable. Thus, it is subject to the appreciation of the observer and the conditions in which the observation is made. Conversely, it can be affected by whether the eyes were kept closed or opened after death and directly by weather conditions.

6.1 At the posterior segment level (Retinal changes)

The assessment of the eye fundus, even in living people, is mainly subjective. Thus, changes seen after death are relatively complex for a forensic pathologist to assess. These have been described since 1920 by Würdermann as an opaque and folded membrane due to retinal infiltration and disorganization, which subsequently stains gray mainly around the optic nerve and the macula; 10–12 hours after death, observing this phenomenon more frequently in young cadavers. Toru Oshima et al. observed the appearance of the retinal fold in 63.3% of corpses, also observed on ocular ultrasound [18]. Death in the prone position was not associated with a postmortem retinal fold, unlike death in the prone position. Although it is a complicated phenomenon to observe and has some limitations, it is difficult to distinguish between postmortem retinal folds and antemortem retinal detachment. The other limitation is corneal opacity which makes it impossible to perform adequate ophthalmoscopy r two hours after death. That is when the cornea begins to cloud. Ocular ultrasonography can be used for noninvasive imaging of postmortem vitreoretinal adhesions [18].

Another phenomenon observed in the retina is the fibrin bridges in the retinal vessels, this segmentation begins 10–15 minutes after death, and in the first three hours, it can be stimulated by rotating the head or exerting pressure on the eyeballs or the thorax.

6.2 Decrease in intraocular pressure

Normal intraocular pressure is mainly determined by aqueous humor: the fluid that fills the anterior and posterior chambers of the eye. Average values range between 10 and 20 mmHg [19]. Some authors have concluded that there is an inverse relationship between the decrease in postmortem intraocular pressure and the time elapsed from death. The longer the postmortem interval, the lower the intraocular pressure, presenting a linear drop over time, at a rate of approximately two mmHg per hour, so it can be a helpful indicator in estimating the early postmortem interval [20].

Measuring intraocular pressure by applanation tonometry is a simple, fast, cheap, and easy method to perform. Although, for now, it cannot accurately determine the time of death of a corpse due to the number of modifying variables, it can be helpful as an additional element to the other cadaveric phenomena for the determination of the postmortem interval, thus having another quantitative and reproducible element that collaborates in the investigation of unwitnessed deaths.

6.3 Sunken eyes

As previously mentioned, eyeball turgidity is the result of keeping intraocular pressure, and pressure, in turn, is caused by intraocular fluids. Therefore, the evaporation of intraocular fluids produces a decrease in intraocular pressure, which is a sign late and persistent. This process has been associated as a factor that generates corneal striae, these being one more sign at the ocular level [18].

6.4 New ocular evaluations in postmortem interval estimation

As technology has progressed, medical science has acquired new methods to increase precision and quantitatively measure changes related to the postmortem interval, such as optical coherence tomography image analysis of the cornea and posterior segment, biometrical analysis of the iris, and histological analysis.

7. Eyeball temperature

It is a relatively complex technique. In 2013, Kaliszan used a high-precision thermometer, with which he inserted a probe in the posterior chamber (vitreous) and another in the rectum to make a comparison [21]. Results showed that it is an excellent method for estimating an early postmortem interval. However, it has several limitations, such as the cadaver's changes according to the environmental temperature and humidity, in addition to the complexity of the measurement technique.

8. Changes in vitreous humor metabolites

This method is not new; there have been studies since 1989 reporting on metabolic changes in the vitreous. This approach was used because the vitreous humor is easy to collect and resistant to deterioration, contamination, and bacterial degradation [22]. To determine metabolites, we must perform a direct aspiration of the eyeball and run an analysis in a specialized laboratory. Metabolites that can be used are sodium, chlorine, calcium, and urea nitrogen. However, one of the primary studied metabolites is potassium, for which a linear concentration relationship, increasing with time after death, of approximately 0.203 mmol per hour has been determined [23]. Vitreous urea nitrogen is also a stable postmortem parameter. It provides information on the homeostasis of electrolyte metabolism. However, these values can be affected by various factors such as environmental temperature, electrolyte imbalances at the time of death, and previous alcohol consumption to death. The standard deviation in various studies is significant [24].

9. Lens alteration

It has been recently described that the lens can change after death. A statistically significant reduction in both absorbance and sphericity has been found, as well as gradual decomposition of the structure and organization of the lens components. The results were corroborated by histologic examination and digital images produced within 96 hours of death [25]. It should be noted that it is a very specialized method, and there is still no research on humans.

10. Optical coherence tomography (OCT)

OCT is an imaging technique based on low coherence interferometry. It allows noncontact tissue to be studied three-dimensionally and in real time. Portable OCT allowed Matteo Nioi et al. to evaluate morphometric changes in the postmortem period's cornea, sclera, and vitreous humor.

In the cornea, studies have found a progressive tendency towards tissue thickening and the progressive formation of waves in the endothelial tissue layer, with increased endothelial reflectivity (Nioi-Napoli sign). Nonetheless, cornea thickness is greatly influenced by factors such as eyelid opening because when the eyes remain open, a rapid reduction in thickness is observed within the first few hours, whereas, when they are closed, this parameter increases progressively [8].

Researchers have also observed a decreased amplitude of the anterior chamber and changes in the iridocorneal angle, corneal edema 6 hours after death, and total loss of corneal epithelium 36 hours after death [8].

OCT changes in the sclera were characterized by hyperreflectivity of the outer layer with physical separation between the sclera and choroids, although studies to determine this phenomenon are still lacking. In the retina, analysis was limited due to pupil size and media opacity (lens and cornea), as previously described.

11. Conclusions

Developing a reliable and easily replicable method for estimating the time since death remains one of forensic medicine's most significant and oldest challenges—the limitations for the practical and daily use of these methods of the essence. Mathematical issues have limited parameters, such as postmortem pupillary diameter and eyeball temperature variations. In contrast, required subjective descriptions mainly limit variations in parameters such as corneal transparency and retinal changes. Regarding lens alterations, they are currently not approved for forensic use, and their evaluation is also highly invasive. The use of computational models is currently limited by the lack of solid data necessary to produce a reliable model; however, the inclusion of ocular phenomena can be helpful as an additional element to the other cadaveric phenomena for determining postmortem interval, thus having quantitative and reproducible elements. Furthermore, eyes are an ideal data source to estimate postmortem interval because of their ease of reach, and some components can be highly predictable. We cannot deny that the enormous and persistent effort to find a solution to this problem has contributed to a better understanding of the macroscopic, microscopic, and molecular changes after death.

Author details

Sandra Vianney Ramírez Ojeda[1*] and Cesar Hernandez Mier[2]

1 School of Medicine, Autonomous University of San Luis Potosí, México, San Luis Potosí, México

2 Law School "Abogado Ponciano Arriaga Leija", Autonomous University of San Luis Potosí, México, San Luis Potosí, México

*Address all correspondence to: vianneyrmzojeda@gmail.com

References

[1] Meurs J, Krap T, Duijst W. Evaluation of postmortem biochemical markers: Completeness of data and assessment of implication in the field. Science & Justice. 2019;**59**(2):177-180. DOI: 10.1016/j.scijus.2018.09.002

[2] Riaz Q, Anwar H, Rizwan H, Phil M. Medico legal importance of post-mortem interval. (An autopsy based study). Ophtalmology. 2016;**4**:92-104

[3] Rafael M. Bañón González y Juan Pedro Hernández del Rincón. "Determinación de la data en el periodo precoz de la muerte. Métodos instrumentals". Revista Española de Medicina Legal. 2010;**36**(2):83-86

[4] Milroy CM. Forensic taphonomy: The postmortem fate of human remains. BMJ. 1999;**319**(7207):458

[5] Lundquist F, Curry AS. Methods of Forensic Science. Vol. 42. London, New York: Interscience Publishers (ed); 1963. pp. 356-367

[6] Swann LM, Forbes SL, Lewis SW. Analytical separations of mammalian decomposition products for forensic science. Analytica Chimica Acta. 2010;**682**(1-2):9-22

[7] Gisbert C. Medicina Legal y Toxicología. Barcelona: Elsevier; 1998. pp. 191-194

[8] Malthotra A, Minja FJ, Crum A, Burrowes D. Ocular anatomy and ross-sectional imaging of the eye. Seminars in Ultrasound, CT, and MR. 2011;**32**(1):2-13

[9] Kanski J. *Oftalmología* Clínica. 9th ed. Glaucoma: Harcourt (ed). pp. 229-203

[10] Moreno C, Fagundez V. Traumatismos oculares: Aspectos médico-legales. Cuadernos de Medicina Forense. 2012;**29**:5-19

[11] Nioi M, Napoli PM, Demontis R, Locci E, Fossarello M, D'Aloja E. Postmortem ocular findings in the optical coherence tomography era: A proof of concept study based on six forensic cases. Diagnostics (Basel). 2021;**11**(3):413

[12] De-Giorgio F, Grassi S, d'Aloja E, Pascali VL. Post-mortem ocular changes and time since death: Scoping review and future perspective. Legal Medicine (Tokyo, Japan). 2021;**50**:101862

[13] Jaafar S, Nokes LD. Examination of the eye as a means to determine the early postmortem period: A review of the literature. Forensic Science International. 1994;**64**(2-3):185-189

[14] Wroblewski BM. Estimation of time of death by eye changes. Forensic Science. 1973;**2**(2):201-205

[15] Koehler K, Sehner S, Riemer M, Gehl A, Raupach T, Anders S. Post-mortem chemical excitability of the iris should not be used for forensic death time diagnosis. International Journal of Legal Medicine. 2018;**132**(6): 1693-1697

[16] Wilson A, Serafin S, Seckiner D, Berry R, Mallett X. Evaluating the utility of time-lapse imaging in the estimation of postmortem interval: An Australian case study. Forensic Science International: Synergy. 2019;**1**:204-210

[17] Oshima T, Yoshikawa H, Ohtani M, Mimasaka S. Examination of postmortem retinal folds: A non-invasive study. Journal of Forensic and Legal Medicine. 2015;**30**:16-20

[18] Lanza M, Laccarino S, Mele L, Carnevale UA, Irregolare C, Lanza A, et al. Intraocular pressure evaluation in healthy eyes and diseased ones using contact and non contact devices. Contact Lens & Anterior Eye. 2016;**39**(2):154-159

[19] Ramírez S, Rangel M, Mier C. Tonometria ocular en pacientes críticos y su comportamiento. Revista Española de Medicina Legal. 2020;**3**:329-336

[20] Kaliszan M. Studies on time of death estimation in the early post mortem period – application of a method based on eyeball temperature measurement to human bodies. Legal Medicine (Tokyo, Japan). 2013;**15**(5):278-282

[21] Coe JI. Vitreous potassium as a measure of the postmortem interval: An historical review and critical evaluation. Forensic Science International. 1989;**42**(3):201-213

[22] Lange N, Swearer S, Sturner WQ. Human postmortem interval estimation from vitreous potassium: An analysis of original data from six different studies. Forensic Science International. 1994;**66**(3):159-174

[23] Ekaterina A, Zelentsova LV, Yanshole OA, Snytnikova VV, et al. Post-mortem changes in the metabolomic compositions of rabbit blood, aqueous and vitreous humors. Metabolomics. 2016;**12**:172

[24] Prieto-Bonete G, Perez-Carceles MD, Luna A. Morphological and histological changes in eye lens: Possible application for estimating postmortem interval. Legal Medicine (Tokyo, Japan). 2015;**17**(6):437-442

[25] Napoli PE, Nioi M, Gabiati L, Laurenzo M, De-Giorgio F, Scorcia V, et al. Repeatability and reproducibility of post-mortem central corneal thickness measurements using a portable optical coherence tomography system in humans: A prospective multicenter study. Scientific Reports. 2020;**10**(1):14508

Chapter 7

Bioethical Issues in Neurorehabilitation

Ivet B. Koleva, Borislav R. Yoshinov, Julieta S. Gerenova, Teodora A. Asenova and Radoslav R. Yoshinov

Abstract

The authors analyze basic bioethical issues, with application in neurorehabilitation clinical practice. We consider traditions of Bulgarian schools of Physical and Rehabilitation Medicine, Physiotherapy and Ergotherapy, related to bioethics. Physical and rehabilitation medicine investigates the effects of the application of natural and preformed physical modalities on the human organism. Neurorehabilitation is an interdisciplinary field - between neurology, neurosurgery and physical medicine. Many principles of the Declaration on bioethics and patients' rights are obligatory in the rehabilitation practice, e.g.: human dignity and human rights, autonomy, consent, equality and equity, non-discrimination and non-stigmatization (for patients with disabilities). Several bioethical topics are important for neurorehabilitation: human research, neuro-ethics, pain management, assisted suicide, euthanasia. We present an analysis of bioethical problems of a clinical case from our neurorehabilitation practice.

Keywords: bioethics, rehabilitation, neurorehabilitation, patient's rights, informed consent, education

1. Introduction

Physical and rehabilitation medicine investigates the effects of the application of natural and preformed physical modalities on the human organism. Neurorehabilitation is an interdisciplinary field - between neurology, neurosurgery and physical medicine. Many principles of Bioethics are obligatory in our rehabilitation and neurorehabilitation practice: human dignity and human rights, autonomy, consent, equality and equity, non-discrimination and non-stigmatization (for patients with disabilities). Several bioethical topics are important for neurorehabilitation: human research, neuro-ethics, pain management, assisted suicide, euthanasia.

2. Rehabilitation, physical medicine, neurorehabilitation

Rehabilitation is a functional therapy, based on a correct functional analysis. Rehabilitation is important element of the treatment of acute and chronic patients and is realized in departments and clinics of hospitals for active care or for long-term care. The rehabilitation process is done by a multi-disciplinary and multi-professional team (medical doctors, nurses, physiotherapists, occupational therapists, psychologists, etc.).

Neurorehabilitation (NR) is an interdisciplinary field - between neurology, neurosurgery and physical medicine.

The rehabilitation is the use of all means for reduction of the impact of disabling and handicapping conditions, and for social integration of the persons with disabilities.

The World Report on Disability of the World Health Organization and World Bank [1] defines the goals of rehabilitation, emphasizing on function: "prevention and slowing the rate of loss of function; improvement, restoration or compensation of lost function; maintenance of current function". Contemporary rehabilitation applies a holistic approach to the patient, based on the International Classification, disability and Health (ICF) [2] and on clinical principles (**Figure 1**).

The rehabilitation process begins with a detailed functional assessment; on this base we formulate the (individual) rehabilitation goals, and we define the rehabilitation program, with evaluation of individual outcomes.

The "Rehabilitation team" includes several medical specialists and health professionals, including the patient and his/her proxy (**Figure 2**).

According the Definition, formulated by the Council of the European Union of Medical Specialists - UEMS [3]: "The medical act encompasses all the professional action, e.g. scientific, teaching, training and educational, clinical and medico-technical steps, performed to promote health and functioning, prevent diseases, provide diagnostic or therapeutic and rehabilitative care to patients, individuals, groups or communities in the framework of the respect of ethical and deontological value. It is the responsibility of, and must always be performed by a registered medical doctor or under his or her direct supervision and/or prescription."

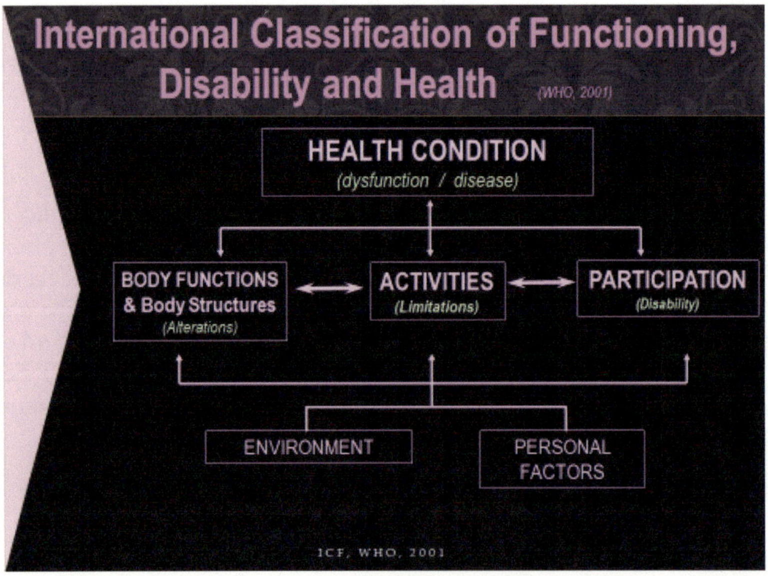

Figure 1.
ICF.

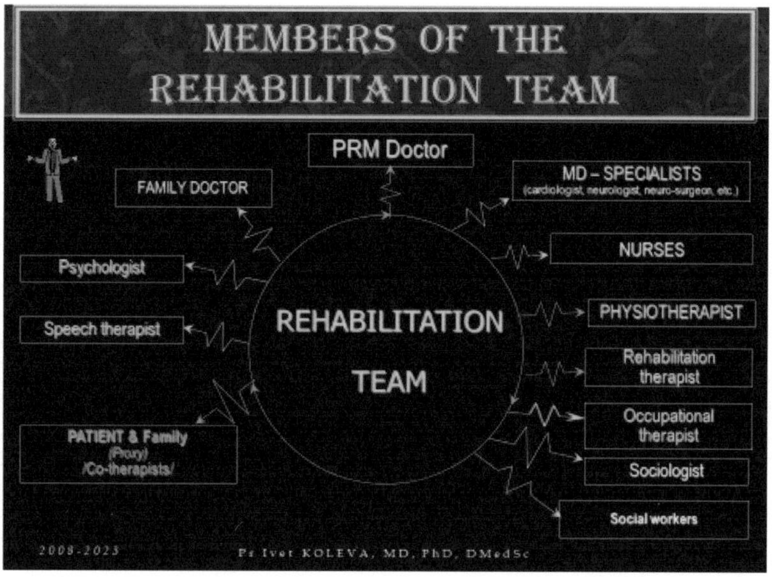

Figure 2.
Members of the rehabilitation team.

According the White Book of the specialty Physical and Rehabilitation Medicine (PRM) and the corresponding definition of the UEMS – PRM Section and Board [4]: PRM is an „independent medical specialty, oriented to the promotion of physical and cognitive functioning, activities (including environment), participation (including quality of life) and changes in personal factors and environment. It is thus responsible for the prevention, diagnosis, treatments and rehabilitation management of people with disabling medical conditions and co-morbidity across all ages."

PRM is a "Medicine of Functioning", focusing on the improvement of individual and social functioning of every patient [5]; so, the application ICF is crucial.

Ultimately, we observe an increasing number of chronic patients with invalidating conditions (predominantly of the nervous, motor and cardio-vascular systems). In NR clinical practice, we have patients with diseases of the central and peripheral nervous system (SNC and PNS). From the SNC conditions, we have patients with: post-stroke hemiparesis, multiple sclerosis, Parkinsonism; brain tumors and cerebral aneurysm (after neurosurgical intervention); traumatic brain injury and traumatic spinal cord injury (with quadriplegia or paraplegia); rare diseases (e.g. Amyotrophic Lateral Sclerosis, Barre-Lieou syndrome). From the group of PNS conditions, we have patients with: cervico-brachial plexopathy and lumbo-sacral radiculopathy, discal hernia (before and after neurosurgery); diabetic polyneuropathy; traumatic injury of peripheral nerves (with radial or peroneal or tibial paresis); Bell's palsy; neuromuscular diseases (e.g. Duchenne muscular dystrophy), etc. All these persons have somato-sensory, motor and/or cognitive dysfunctions and deficits; including: deficits in voluntary movements and postural adaptation, problems of the motor planning and coordination, functional ability and autonomy in activities in daily living (ADL) (**Figure 3**). Therefore, our patients need complex rehabilitation programs, with emphasis on functional recovery and amelioration of the autonomy in everyday life. In this process, we use different natural and preformed physical modalities. In clinical rehabilitation practice, we apply a holistic and patient-centered approach [4].

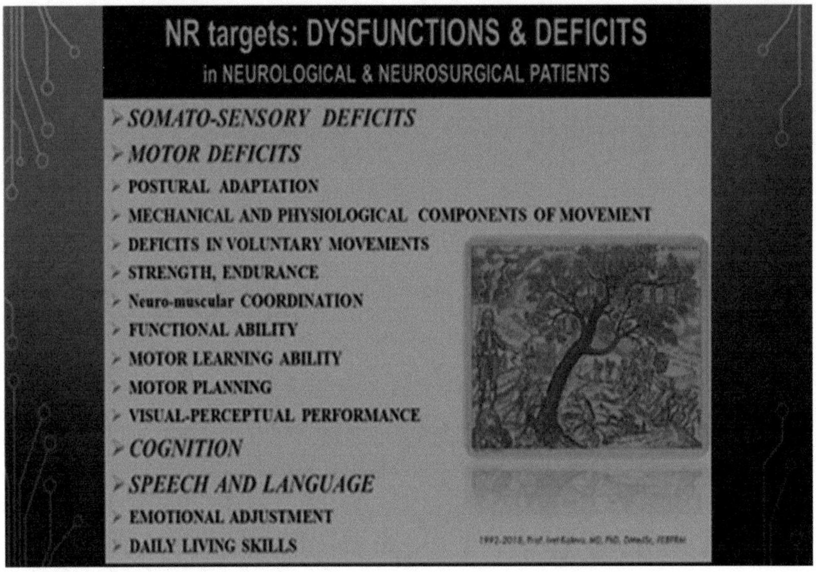

Figure 3.
Frequent dysfunctions and deficits in NR clinical practice.

The diagnosis in PRM is a combination of the medical diagnosis, based on the International Classification of Diseases (ICD), and a specific functional evaluation, based on the International Classification of Functioning, Disability and Health (ICF). Interventions in PRM are programed by the PRM physicians and are provided by the members of the rehabilitation team. We apply medicines, physical therapy, ergotherapy (occupational therapy), procedures with different natural and preformed physical factors, patient education. The principle of this complex program or rehabilitation "puzzle' is presented in **Figure 4**.

Results of PRM interventions currently show reduction of impairments in body functions and activity limitations, influence on participation restrictions, and also reduction in costs, as well as decrease in mortality for certain groups of patients.

The goal of PRM is physical prevention, treatment by physical factors, and rehabilitation of physical or psychical dysfunction.

The medical doctors – PRM specialists are engaged in the clinical management of neurological and neurosurgical, rheumatological and traumatological, cardiological and cardio-surgical patients.

The Neurorehabilitation (NR) algorithm includes detailed functional assessment (based on ICD and ICF) and a therapeutic program of physical factors (movement, activities, mineral waters, electric currents, etc.). The "rehabilitation puzzle" (**Figures 4** and **5**) is a synergic combination of various physical modalities:

- Natural physical factors: water (mineral baths), air (air baths), sun (sun baths), exercises (active, passive, against gravity, contra resistance), massage (manual, vibration, etc.), manual therapy techniques (traction, mobilization, and manipulation); occupational therapy (work and activities);

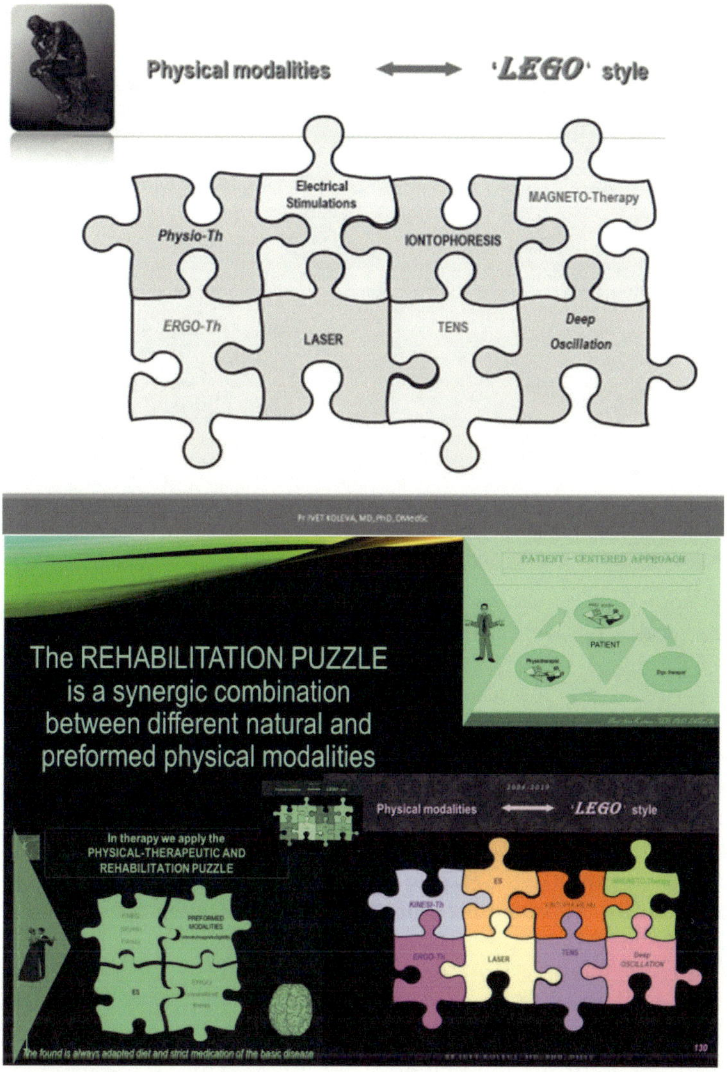

Figure 4.
The "rehabilitation puzzle", applied in PRM practice.

- Pre-formed physical modalities: electric currents (low, middle and high frequency currents), electro-static field (deep oscillation); light (infrared, visible and ultra-violet light beams; Laser), magnetic field, ultra-sound, etc.).

Physical and rehabilitation medicine investigates the effects of the application of natural and preformed physical modalities on the human organism.

The common NR-algorithm includes one or two pre-formed physical modalities (electrotherapy, magnetotherapy, phototherapy, ultrasound therapy), one thermo- or cryo-agent, two or three physiotherapeutic and ergotherapeutic procedures (including analytic exercises, post-isometric relaxation, stretching techniques, massage, training in activities of daily living, etc.).

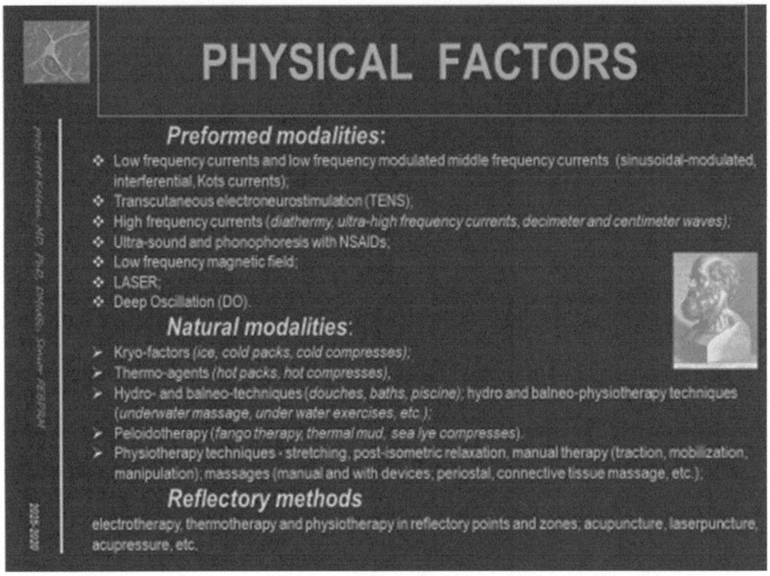

Figure 5.
Physical modalities (physical factors).

3. Ethics, bioethics, and neurorehabilitation

3.1 Ethics and bioethics

Ethics is based on morality, answering the "classical" questions: what is right or wrong, what is just or unjust. The Code of Ethics includes: integrity, objectivity, honesty, moral values, responsibility, professional competence, confidentiality, professional behavior [6].

Bioethics is a expansion of the principal idea of the Hippocratic Oath "Primum non nocere" (the concept of "First Do Not Harm") for all medical doctors and health professionals. According to definitions, bioethics is the "study of ethical issues arising from advances in biology and medicine" [7, 8]. It is also moral discernment in medical policy and practice. Bioethics is a field of study and professional practice, based on ethical principles. It includes the study of values ("ordinary ethics") in relation to various medical and biological scientific fields [6, 7]. Bioethics derives from the Greek words bios (life) and ethos (behavior, moral nature). In 1926, Fritz Jahr applied this noun in an article about a "bioethical imperative" concerning the routine of usage of animals and plants in scientific research. In 1970, the American biochemist Van Rensselaer Potter applied the term and founded the global ethics.

Every medical doctor or health professional estimates the patients' rights. In bioethics, we consider rights as the basic normative rules according to ethical theory. In rehabilitation practice, patients' rights include rights related to treatment and safety, access to care and choice of care, participation in decision-making process, seek for a second opinion, compassionate palliative care and end-of-life care. For example, the right to appropriate medical care; right to informed consent; right to access information and medical record; right to privacy and confidentiality; right of choice of the physician and hospital; right to refuse diagnostics and treatment, right to decline participation in research; right to social contacts.

The Universal Declaration on bioethics and human rights [8], adopted by the General conference of UNESCO (in 2005), formulated the principles of bioethics (**Figure 6**). From the list of 15 principles, the most important for the NR practice remain: human dignity and human rights, benefit and harm, autonomy and individual responsibility; consent, privacy and confidentiality; equality, justice and equity; non-discrimination and non-stigmatization. Some patients in psychiatric, pediatric or geriatric rehabilitation, are persons without the capacity to consent, and for them the principle of respect for human vulnerability and personal integrity is essential. The principles of social responsibility and sharing of benefits are applied in many rehabilitation patients.

The list of topics concerning bioethics [9–11] covers many areas of medicine and health care (**Figure** 7). For NR- practice, the most important are: Human research, Neuroethics, Disability, Pain management, Assisted suicide and Euthanasia.

3.2 Medical ethics

Medical ethics is the application of moral values in medicine and healthcare.

In the field of medical ethics, we note the central locus of the Declaration of Geneva, adopted by the Second General Assembly of the World Medical Association in 1948, last revised in 2017 [12]. This Declaration includes the physicians' pledge upon honor for dedication "to the service of humanity", and is known as the "Modern Hippocratic Oath".

The World Medical Association (WMA) has established the International Code of Medical Ethics [13], adopted by the General Assembly of WMA in London in 1949, last revision in 2022. The Code states professional duties of medical doctors: principles of the physicians' behavior and conduct, promotion of patient's health and well-being, competent and qualitative care of patients in clinical practice. The Code states too principles of the physicians' comportment to colleagues, to health professionals,

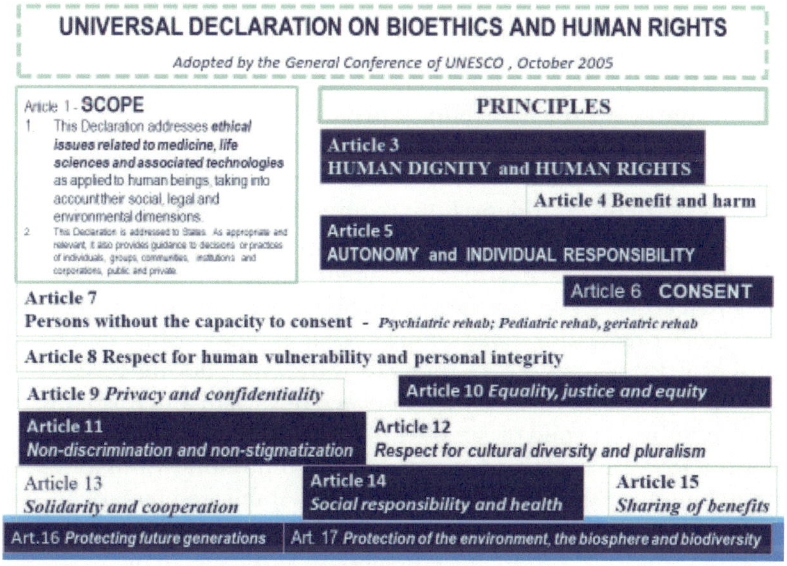

Figure 6.
Universal declaration on bioethics and human rights, 2005.

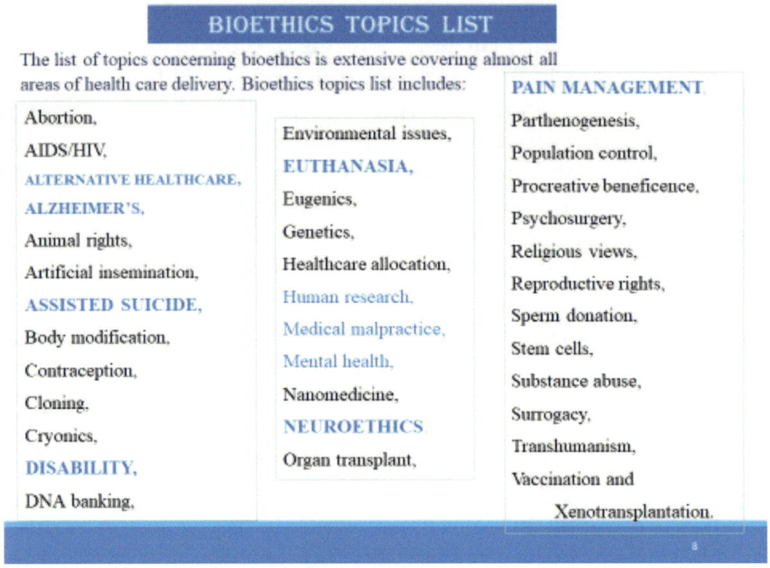

Figure 7.
Bioethics topics list.

to students, and to society. The Code is applied everywhere: in medical centers and in hospitals (emergency, acute departments, rehabilitation wards).

Common ethical principles, valid for every field of medicine, include: honesty, accuracy of actions, morality, equality, respect for rights, autonomy, integrity and adherence to the law, confidentiality, authenticity, responsibility, transparency [14].

These basic ethical principles are developed in the Ethics Manual of the American College of Physicians (ACP), first published in 1984 [15, 16]. The last (seventh) edition of 2018 introduced various new and expanded sections on some modern themes, as follows: Electronic communications, Telemedicine ethics, On-line professionalism, Internet and social media research. The Manual facilitates the decision-making in some cases presenting ethical dilemmas [17].

The Manual comments the basic ethical principles [17]: beneficence and non-maleficence, respect for patient's autonomy, and justice. Various other ethical issues are discussed: professionalism of the medical doctor, communication between the physician and the patient; confidentiality; requirements for the medical record (paper or electronic); informed decision-making and consent. Special attention is paid to some "difficult" situations, as: health-care system catastrophes (infections, natural disasters, terrorist attacks); or cases of provided medical care to persons, proxy to the physician (with preexisting close nonprofessional relationship, or a reporting relationship), or VIPs; palliative care and end-of-life (incl. do-not-resuscitate order, euthanasia); cases of sexual involvement between physician and former patients; gifts from patients or industry; solid organ transplantation; etc.

Specific situations are explained, e.g. electronic communications and euthanasia.

Electronic communications are permitted in an established patient-physician relationship and they can be applied only with patient consent. A telemedicine encounter must begin with steps for creation of a connection, as during an in-person visit.

Most medical organizations do not support physician-assisted suicide and euthanasia. Ten American states and the District of Columbia have legalized the practice of physician-assisted suicide in USA [18]. The situation in Europe is similar: some countries accept (as Switzerland, Spain, Belgium, Netherlands); others do not agree with the physician-assisted suicide. This type of Death at Dignitas is for the moment not entirely accepted.

3.3 Bioethical principles in neurorehabilitation

Bioethical principles, important for NR, are: beneficence and non-maleficence (work for people's welfare and reduction of harm: personal, social, organizational); fidelity and responsibility (and professional transparency); justice (equal access to medical care, without discrimination and biases) [14].

Many principles of the Universal Declaration on Bioethics and Human rights of UNESCO are obligatory in rehabilitation practice: human dignity and human rights, autonomy and individual responsibility, informed consent, equality and equity, non-discrimination and non-stigmatization (for patients with disabilities), social responsibility [8].

From the list of bioethical topics, the most important issues for NR are: human research, neuro-ethics, pain management, assisted suicide, euthanasia.

Many patients in NR-clinical practice have reduced autonomy and disability; they require assistive technologies, home adaptations, and complex pain management. In terminal cases, we have ethical problems and dilemmas (especially informed consent and the right to euthanasia).

Important bioethical aspects are the connections between the patient and the NR team; and the interactions between different members of the multi-professional multi-disciplinary NR team.

As in every hospital, the Informed consent is an obligatory rule in NR departments and clinics. Informed consent is the processus of instruction of the patient (by the health provider) about the benefits, risks and alternatives of the diagnostic or therapeutic procedures. In case of emergency or incompetence of the patient (in pediatric and geriatric rehabilitation, or in case of altered conscience), the informed consent is by the patient's proxy.

Actually, in NR we apply largely Information and Communication Technologies (ICT): robotic rehabilitation with virtual reality; grasp and gait training with Exoskeletons, systems Tyro-motion and Lokomat, etc. Computer-based NR is very expensive, and this states the problem of equal access of all patients to contemporaneous (including ICT-based) methods for diagnostics and treatment.

3.4 Patients' rights in neurorehabilitation

The Declaration of Lisbon (1981, last revision in 2015) defines the basic patient's rights [19]: right to medical care of good quality, right to freedom of choice, right to self-determination, right to information, right to confidentiality, right to health education, right to dignity, right to religious assistance.

Every physician must always act in the patient's best interest, even in cases of unconscious or legally incompetent patient (altered brain functioning or loss of consciousness, consequence of traumatic brain injury, concussion or psychiatric condition). In this situation, the medical doctor necessitates the decision of the patient's official representative. Diagnostic or therapeutic procedures against the patient's will can be realized only in exceptional cases, in compliance to the principles of medical ethics.

In a previous publication [20], we analyzed the opinion on ethical issues of academic staffs, rehabilitation staffs and patients from acute and long-term rehabilitation departments. Our results demonstrated the close relationship between the PRM-clinical practice and many principles of the Universal Declaration on Bioethics and some typical bioethical topics, especially human research, neuroethics, pain management, euthanasia. From the Declaration on Bioethics and Human Rights of UNESCO (2005) the most important for NR are: human dignity and human rights, autonomy; informed consent, persons without the capacity to consent (psychiatric rehabilitation; pediatric rehabilitation, geriatric rehabilitation); equality and equity; non-discrimination and non-stigmatization (for patients with disability). For the *academic staff in PRM* and for the *staff of PRM Clinics,* the most important are: Patient's consent, Autonomy, Human dignity, Research. The Research is important only for the academic staff. All members of the inter-professional and interdisciplinary rehabilitation team consider necessary the formulation of the fields of competence and responsibility of every team member. *Patients of early rehabilitation department* consider as most relevant pain management, rights to contemporary rehabilitation techniques and ICT-based devices, right to use modern technical aids, and right to choose a concrete medical doctor and therapist. The most significant items for *patients in chronic phase* (long-term care and rehabilitation) were: autonomy, home adaptation, rights to receive proper information, right to apply contemporaneous treatment methods and devices. Young patients (*age-groups 25 to 55 years)* consider crucial the right of modern methods of rehabilitation, as virtual reality, robots and neuro-robots. For p*atients and staff of geriatric rehabilitation department* the most important are the rights to information (concerning the prognosis), the pain management, the right of technical aids and home adaptations, the right of active or passive euthanasia.

A collective of several academics of Canadian Universities (McGill University, McMaster University, Montreal University, Ottawa University) investigated the problem of *patient's autonomy*, analyzing results of 16 empirical reports, 17 case studies and 30 theoretical papers [21]. The authors focused on four approaches for responding to patient autonomy: supporting, promoting, respecting and advocating [21]. Their conclusions coincide with the opinion on patients' autonomy of our academic staff and the rehabilitation staff of PRM Departments of early and chronic stage. Autonomy is considered as significant issue for our patients of clinics of long-term care and rehabilitation.

Patients' autonomy in decision-making is underlined as an important dilemma by staffs of spinal cord injury (SCI) rehabilitation department in developing world, according small group discussions in three medical conferences [22]. In low-income and lower-middle-income countries, many other ethical problems are present, e.g. lack of insurance for SCI rehabilitation and numerous financial challenges [22].

Ghostal et al. [23] discuss problems of *cancer-related communication*. Oncologic patients prefer the on time disclosure of diagnosis and prognosis, allowing for the necessity of planning consecutive steps for their families [23]. Our patients of chronic stage rehabilitation departments consider too the right to receive adequate information as early as possible.

We observed some parallels between concerns of our patients and staff of geriatric rehabilitation department and opinions of *patients of a department of palliative care*, according an article of Chaturvedi [24]. Our results include: rights to information (and prognosis), to pain management, to receive technical aids and home adaptations, right to dignity and right of active or passive euthanasia. Patients and staff in palliative care settings consider important the following themes: use of oral morphine for pain relief, spiritual care, lack of adequate palliative care services, and palliative care education [24]. Pain management is an important issue for our patients of the early rehabilitation department.

3.5 Bioethical issues in elderly patients in neurorehabilitation

In October 2022 in Berlin, Germany, the World Medical Association accepted a Declaration on Discrimination against elderly individuals within healthcare settings [25]. The Declaration of Berlin recommends to eliminate all forms of discrimination due to health and age. The need for a holistic approach in elderly is discussed. The Declaration commends to medical doctors include to provide healthcare of scientific and human quality according to good medical practice to all patients, without any discrimination.

3.6 Bioethical issues in the field of research in neurorehabilitation

The basic principles of the Ethics of Research are explained in the "Belmont Report: Ethical Principles and Guidelines for Research Involving Human Subjects" [26]. These three principles are valid in rehabilitation and neurorehabilitation: respect for persons, beneficence and non-maleficence and justice. The first principle of Respect for persons includes the requirement to recognize autonomy of patients and the obligation to defend persons with reduced autonomy. The second principle of beneficence and non-maleficence is based on the Hippocratic aphorism of "First, do not harm" and includes the responsibility to assure the well-being of patients. The third principle of Justice assure the equal attitude to all patients. Practical applications of these principles include the Informed consent, the assessment of risks and benefits, and the selection of subjects for investigations.

Research in NR are suborned to the 10 principles for investigation, formulated in the Nuremberg Code [27], with special consideration to the voluntary informed consent of every participant.

The same principles are mentioned in the Seventh Edition of the Ethics Manual of the American College of Physicians (ACP), elaborated by the Ethics, Professionalism and Human Rights Committee (EPHRC) [17]. The first principle of respect for persons is transformed into respect for patient autonomy, explained as "duty to protect and foster a patient's free, uncoerced choices". The second principle of beneficence is divided into beneficence and non-maleficence. Beneficence is explained as "duty to promote good and act in the best interest of the patient". The non-maleficence is described as "duty to do no harm to the patient". The third principle of Justice is defined as "equitable distribution of the life-enhancing opportunities afforded by health care".

The same Ethics Manual of the ACP postulates the requirement of a Decision from an Institutional Review Board (IRB) for every research. This step assures the protection of the human subjects, an acceptable benefit-risk ration, adequate informed consent process and confidentiality safety.

The Declaration of Helsinki of the World Medical Association clarifies the Ethical principles for medical research, involving human subjects [28]. The document is adopted by the WMA General Assembly in Helsinki in 1964 and is amended by next general assemblies, last one in 2013. According this Declaration the duty of medical doctors is to protect the life and health, to respect the dignity and integrity, to esteem the privacy, and confidentiality of personal information of research subjects.

An analysis of risks, burdens and benefits is done. Special attention is paid to privacy and confidentiality, informed consent, use of placebo, etc.

3.7 Bioethics and education in neurorehabilitation

The title "doctor" comes from Latin: "*docere*" means "to teach", therefore physicians are responsible to teach colleagues and patients. To share knowledge and information includes teaching clinical skills and reporting results of scientific research to other physicians, medical students and trainees. Patient education is part of the doctors' duties to society [14, 17].

The World Federation for Medical Education (WFME) has elaborated on global standards for basic medical education (last update 2020) [29]. Standards for basic medical education include curriculum content and structure, organization, educational resources, requirements for the academic staff, process of admission of students. The education of future physicians is discussed in many publications [30].

In 2021, WFME published the "Standards for distributed and distance learning in medical education" [31]. Different forms of learning are debated: distance learning, distributed learning, online learning, e-learning, virtual learning, and flexible learning. The requirements for the design of a typical course is presented [31].

For a post-graduate course in neurorehabilitation (during long-life-learning of medical doctors – specialists and trainees in PRM, and of health professionals), we made a curriculum [32], including some principal educational modules, as follows: neuroanatomy, neurophysiology, modern methods of NR, etc. The theoretical part was done online, with power-point presentations, electronic books [33] and videos. The practical part must be face-to-face to the patients. In exceptional circumstances (COVID-pandemic), we used videos with case studies of real or virtual patients. The assessment of learners' competences was done using tests (some of them – online) and a practical exam (face-to-face to a patient). The decision-making process is easier in case of traditional learning (with a patient). During the COVID-pandemic, we prepared and realized educational courses on the topics "Rehabilitation in SARS-CoV-2" [34] and "ICT-based Neurorehabilitation in Neuro-COVID" [35].

4. Case report with ethical dilemmas

4.1 Clinical case presentation

4.1.1 General case presentation

We present a patient, who is a 23-years-old male with inferior paraplegia, due to a cranio-cerebral and severe spinal cord traumatic injury. The trauma is a consequence of an occupational accident – fall from a height of about 15 meters, from a construction site.

4.1.2 Medical dimension

The patient had trauma of the head, chest, spine and pelvis. MRI-data of polyfragmentary fracture of the bodies of thoracic vertebral bodies Th7 and Th8, with bone fragments in the spinal cord and anatomic discontinuity in the thoracic myelon, fracture of the transversal processes of Th4-Th8 vertebrae. Diagnosed right hemothorax; pneumothorax, multiple fractures of the dorsal part of the 4th to the 7th right ribs, dorsally; fractures of the scapula and the right acetabulum.

During the first month, intensive care and resuscitation, ventilator support and neuro-surgical intervention were performed – decompression of the thoracic spinal cord, with subsequent transpedicular osteosynthesis (**Figure 8**). During the operation, a communication between the hemothorax and the thoracic spine was observed.

On the admission at the Hospital for Long-term care and Rehabilitation – Department of Physical and Rehabilitation Medicine (PRM), we observed an inferior central paraplegia with complete anesthesia in lower extremities, with a sensory level Th11 on the right side and Th12 on the left side.

During the stay in the PRM-Department (for about 4 weeks), a verticalization was done; every day a NR-complex was conducted, including physiotherapy (analytic exercises, balance training), occupational therapy (ADL training, gait training with a walker, then with crutches), and preformed physical modalities (electrical stimulations for feet extensors; lasertherapy for an intergluteal decubital wound of grade 1–2).

4.1.2.1 Ethical problem 1

The in-patient rehabilitation is covered by the National insurance funds in our country only for a stay period of 7 to 10 days, the remaining days must be paid by the patient. However, the patient's needs require at least 3 months of active rehabilitation in a hospital setting.

4.1.2.2 Ethical problem 2

A NR-course of 10 procedures of robotic neurorehabilitation is also offered; but this is a paid procedure (and quite expensive). The costs are high and not covered by the National insurance funds.

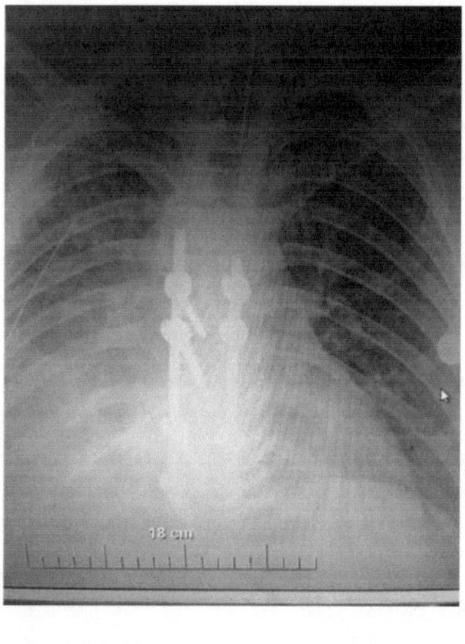

Figure 8.
Transpedicular stabilization of the thoracic spine.

4.1.2.3 Ethical problem 3

It is a well-known fact, that the medical specialists and the health professionals have the duty to tell the truth to their patients. Access to information is an inalienable human right (and patient's right, of course). However, the patient must be conditioned to realize and accept the truth. Often, in such situations, we observe the phenomenon of "difficult" or "delayed" acceptance of the "new" situation – paraplegia, in this case. The patient can pass through phases of: denial, realization, depression, despair, resignation.

The prognosis of our patient with standard treatment is "stabilization" of the inferior paraplegia and autonomy with a wheelchair. We explained the scenario to the patient's parents (accompanying him at this moment). At the insistence of the mother and father, and with the advice of our neuropsychologist and after a psychiatric consultation, we delayed the communication of the full prognosis to the patient for about 2 weeks, as he still had some residual cognitive impairment and emotional instability due to the traumatic brain injury (TBI). The initial reaction of the patient to the accident imposed the necessity of consultation by a psychiatrist, systematic antidepressant therapy and psychotherapy.

There is no guarantee of the recovery of paraplegia in traumatic spinal cord injury (SCI). Partial reduction is possible and transformation into paraparesis, but only in case of active rehabilitation.

4.1.2.4 Ethical problem 4

In the context of modern communication channels, patients and his proxy have access to information for different types of "miraculous recovery". Patient and his family asked us about the possibility of stem cells transplantation. We answered sincerely that some authors consider this operation effective, but without sufficient data, according to the requirements of the evidence-based medicine. In some clinics (but not in our country) this expensive operation is performed, but without guarantees. In cases of professionally performed operation, no negative effects are expected. The final decision is ultimately up to the patient and the family.

4.1.3 Nursing dimension

At the beginning of the stay, the patient presented subfebrility, due to urinary tract infection. Many measures were initiated: catheter replacement, catheter flushes, antibiotic treatment for about 10 days, with periodical sterile urine investigations.

Due to the persistent bed rest, a decubital wound was developed. Many decubitus prevention measures were placed: anti-decubital mattress, back skin inspections, wound dressings.

On several occasions, sedatives and analgesics had to be given.

The patient was accompanied by family members (his mother and father took turns to accompany him). No volunteer assistance was needed.

4.1.4 Functional assessment and neurorehabilitation dimension

We realized some measures for prevention of the consequences of the prolonged bed rest: position treatment (gradual lifting of the upper trunk), passive exercises for lower extremities, including 'muscle pumps' (ankle flexion and extension), balance training in a sitting position. In the complex NR program we included elements of physiotherapy, massage, ergotherapy (occupational therapy), preformed physical modalities (electrical stimulations, laser).

4.2 Patient's views. Social dimension. Organizational dimension

The ethical principle of justice must be respected.

The dignity of the patient and his rights must be esteemed.

4.2.1 Patient's opinions and social dimension

The patient accepted the prognosis (inferior paraparesis or paraplegia), but for him this partial or complete loss of mobility in lower limbs is a problem. Until the trauma, he was physically active. His profession is based on physical activity – he is master-builder. In the future, he must do a professional re-orientation and choose a profession not requiring physical load and possible in a sitting position.

Until the moment of the accident, the patient does not belong to a religious community. At the moment of his transfer to the rehabilitation clinic, the life of the patient is no longer in danger. There is no need for a priest.

The consequences of the trauma are quite serious – both in terms of social and professional engagement, and in terms of remuneration.

We counseled the patient and his parents to seek a professional advice from a lawyer, specialist in labor law, as this was an accident at work. Financial security is important both to carry out the rehabilitation process and to ensure a minimal standard of life in the future.

During the stay at the rehabilitation ward, his girlfriend visited the patient once (no marriage, no children).

The effects of the cranial and spinal cord trauma are difficult for every person to overcome. However, they are especially difficult for a young person, living outside the capital.

4.2.2 Organizational dimension

The bioethical principle of equality, justice and fairness must be respected.

All patient's rights are esteemed: right to quality health services; right to sufficient information with the view of informed consent and decisions concerning the future treatment and rehabilitation; right to access any medical information; right to confidentiality; right to personal dignity; right to self-determination.

4.3 Patient's autonomy. Informed consent

The ethical principle of respect for autonomy is respected. During his stay, the patient was informed in details about his condition and prognosis. Every diagnostic and therapeutic method was explained explicitly to the patient, with existing options to accept or to deny the respective procedure. We need the signed informed consent of the patient at the entry, and before every diagnostic or therapeutic procedure.

In rehabilitation, the active participation of the patient and his family is very important. We stimulated the patient's personal responsibility. The members of the family are treated as co-therapists.

4.4 Responsibility of medical specialists and health professionals

The patient received the exact medications in the right doses, the exact rehabilitation procedures – at precisely defined dosages.

During the daily visits and the weekly main visit, the opinions of the individual members of the medical team (neurologist, PRM-doctor, urologist, etc.) were commented on, as well as the opinions of different health professionals (nurses, physiotherapists, occupational therapists). Practically, the patient and his parents participated as listeners during these discussions, and also as active members of the rehabilitation team. We believe that such discussions should take place with the majority of patients. All medical specialists and health professionals treat confidential information responsibly (with confidentiality).

Rehabilitation patients need a care from an extended multi-professional and multi-disciplinary rehabilitation team, including: doctors – specialists (in Neurology, Orthopedics and Traumatology, Cardiology, Urology, Pulmology, Rheumatology, Psychiatry, etc.); nurses; therapists (physiotherapists, occupational therapists), neuro-psychologist, clinical psychologist; social worker; jurist.

4.5 Decision-making. Special circumstances

4.5.1 Decision-making

In practice, on the admission to a hospital for long-term care and rehabilitation, the patient is informed about the necessary diagnostic and therapeutic techniques. The signature of an informed consent is obligatory at the entry and before any procedure. In case of patient's incompetence, suggested by a neuro-psychologist and diagnosed by a physician – specialist in psychiatry, the decision can be made by the patient's proxy (in this case –his parents).

On the issue of stem cell transplantation, we informed the patient and relatives of the possible risks of surgery. The patient and his family have to decide. The medical and paramedical staff must respect their decision and choice. We are obliged to provide all available medical information – for and against.

4.5.2 Special conditions

During the first two weeks of his hospital stay, our patient had some cognitive dysfunctions and psycho-emotional lability. Therefore, we decided to consider his parents' request and the psychologist's advice to delay the full communication of the prospects to the patient. We informed on time the mother and father of the prognosis, in 2 weeks – we described the "full truth" to the patient. The emotional reaction of the patient was development of a depressive state (suggested by our psychologist and diagnosed by a psychiatrist). In this situation we were obliged to include anti-depressive medication and psychotherapeutic course.

4.6 Right to modern therapeutic methods

Every patient has the right to be treated with contemporaneous methods. The problem is that some modern procedures are very expensive and they are not

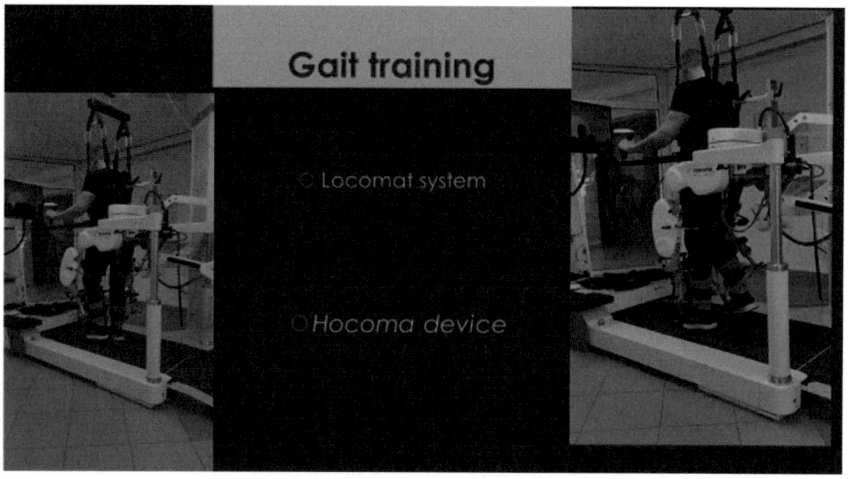

Figure 9.
Robotic neurorehabilitation.

covered by the National health insurance funds. Therefore, the patient must pay for this.

Finally, we find the possibility to obtain the necessary funds from a benevolent organization and this young man received the full possibility to receive robotic rehabilitation, using neurorobots - the device Lokomat of Hocoma (**Figure 9**).

4.7 Prevention of complications

The possible complications in quadriplegia and paraplegia due to TBI and SCI include: deep vein thrombosis, pulmonary thromboembolism, urinary infections, decubital wounds, muscle and joint contractures, arterial hypotonia and orthostatic hypotension, etc.

We made periodical observations and tests, for diagnostic of the early stages of possible complications.

4.8 Right to assistive technologies and to home adaptations

The patient needs assistive technologies and home adaptations, due to the prognosis – spastic paraplegia or paraparesis. The necessary technical aids in this case are: wheelchair, crutches, eventually – canes (**Figure 10**). The minimum home adaptations include: wheelchair ramp, adaptations in the bathroom and in toilet (**Figure 11**).

Part of these technical aids and home adaptations can be assured by the social security funds.

5. Conclusion

Bioethics is an important link between rehabilitation and human values.

Bioethics principles are important element in the everyday clinical practice of neurorehabilitation.

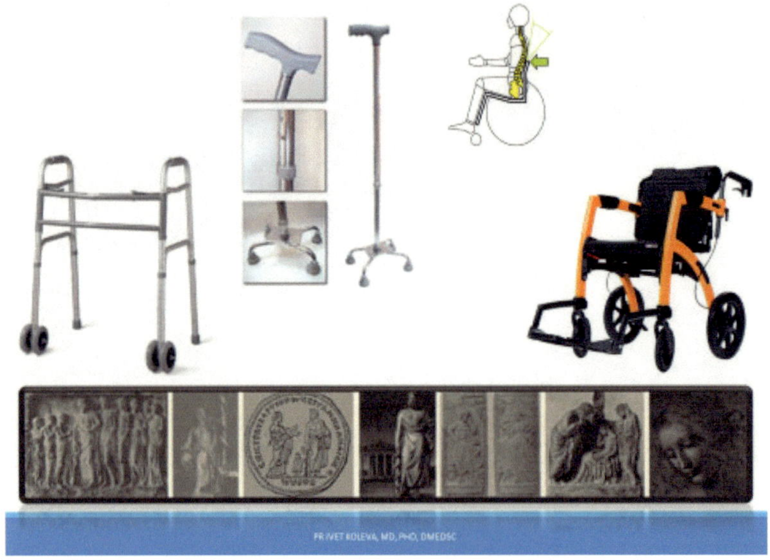

Figurc 10.
Technical aids.

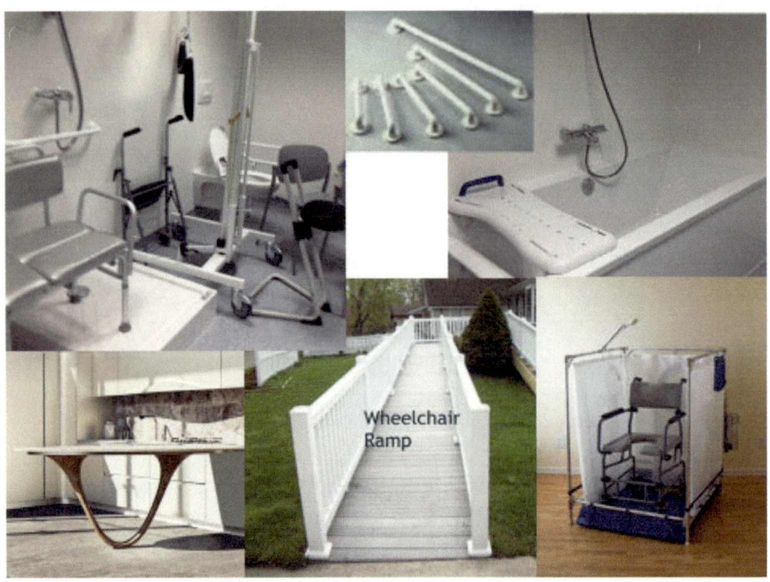

Figure 11.
Home adaptations.

Every member of the multi-professional and multi-disciplinary rehabilitation team must be informed about his duty to consider bioethical laws and patients' rights.

Conflict of interest

The authors declare no conflict of interest.

List of acronyms and abbreviations

ACP	American College of Physicians
ADL	Activities of daily living
COVID	Corona virus disease
EPHRC	Ethics, Professionalism and Human Rights Committee
ICD	International Classification of Diseases
ICF	International Classification of Functioning, Disability and Health
ICT	Information and Communication Technologies
MRI	Magnetic Resonance Imagery
NR	Neurorehabilitation
PRM	Physical and rehabilitation medicine
SCI	Spinal Cord Injury
TBI	Traumatic Brain Injury
UEMS	Union of European Medical Specialists
WHO	World Health Organization
WFME	World Federation for Medical Education
WMA	World Medical Association

Author details

Ivet B. Koleva[1,2,3]*, Borislav R. Yoshinov[4], Julieta S. Gerenova[1], Teodora A. Asenova[4] and Radoslav R. Yoshinov[5]

1 Medical University of Sofia, Bulgaria

2 Specialized Hospital for Long-Term Care and Rehabilitation "Serdika" with Medical Center for Robotic Neurorehabilitation "ReGo", Sofia, Bulgaria

3 Physical Medicine Department, National Heart Hospital, Sofia, Bulgaria

4 Medical Faculty of Sofia University, Sofia, Bulgaria

5 University for Library Studies and Information Technologies, Sofia, Bulgaria

*Address all correspondence to: dr.yvette.5@gmail.com

References

[1] World Health Organization. World Report on Disability. [Internet]. Available from: https://www.who.int/publications-detail/world-report-on-disability [Accessed: May 15, 2012]

[2] World Health Organization. International Classification of Functioning, Disability and Health: ICF. Geneva: WHO; 2001

[3] European Union of Medical Specialists. European Definition of Medical Act. Meeting in Munich [Internet]. 2005. Available from: http://www.uems-slm.org/uems/index.php?id=26 [Accessed: May 15, 2012]

[4] Gutenbrunner C, Ward AB, Chamberlain MA. White book on physical and rehabilitation medicine (PRM) in Europe. Produced by the section of PRM, Union Européenne des médecins spécialistes (UEMS), European board of PRM and académie Européenne de médecine de réadaptation in conjunction with European society for PRM. Produced 2006. Journal of Rehabilitation Medicine. 2007;**39**:1-48. DOI: 10.2340/16501977-0028

[5] European Physical and Rehabilitation Medicine Bodies Alliance. White Book on Physical and Rehabilitation Medicine (PRM) in Europe. Chapter 7. The clinical field of competence: PRM in practice. European Journal of Physics Rehabilitation Medicine. 2018;**54**(2):230-260. DOI: 10.23736/S1973-9087.18.05151-1

[6] Ten Have H. Global Bioethics: An Introduction. London: Routledge; 2016

[7] Engelhardt TH, editor. Global Bioethics: The Collapse of Consensus. Salem: M&M Scrivener Press; 2006

[8] UNESCO. Bioethics. E-book. Sofia: UNESCO; 2018. p. 70

[9] Mitchell CB, Pellegrino E, Elshtain JB, Kilner J, Rae S. Biotechnology and the Human Good. Washington, DC: Georgetown University Press; 2007

[10] Bennett B, editor. Health, Rights, and Globalisation. Surrey, UK: Ashgate; 2006

[11] Cherry M, Peppin JF. Regional Perspectives in Bioethics. Annals of Bioethics. Lisse, The Netherlands: Swets & Zuietlinger; 2003

[12] World Medical Association. Declaration of Geneva [Internet]. Available from: www.wma.net/what-we-do/medical-ethics/declaration-of-geneva/ [Accessed: May 05, 2023]

[13] World Medical Association. WMA international code of medical ethics [Internet]. Available from: www.wma.net/what-we-do/medical-ethics/ [Accessed: May 05, 2023]

[14] World Medical Association. Medical Ethics Manual. 3rd edition 2015 [Internet]. Available from: www.wma.net/wp-content/uploads/2016/11/Ethics_manual_3rd_Nov2015_en.pdf [Accessed: May 05, 2023]

[15] American College of Physicians Ethics Manual. Part 1: History; the patient; other physicians. American College of Physicians. Annals of Internal Medicine. 1989;**111**:245-252

[16] American College of Physicians Ethics Manual. Part 2: The physician and society; research; life-sustaining treatment; other issues. American College of Physicians. Annals of Internal Medicine. 1989;**111**:327-335

[17] Sulmasy LS, Bledsoe TA, for the ACP Ethics, Professionalism and Human Rights Committee. American College of Physicians Ethics Manual. Seventh edition. Annals of Internal Medicine. 15 Jan 2019;**170**(2_Suppl):S1-S32. DOI: 10.7326/M18-2160. PMID: 30641552

[18] Sulmasy LS, Mueller PS for the Ethics, Professionalism and Human Rights Committee of the American College of Physicians. Ethics and the legalization of physician-assisted suicide: An American college of physicians position paper. Annals of Internal Medicine. 2017;**167**(8):576-578. DOI: 10.7326/M17-0938

[19] World Medical Association. WMA Declaration of Lisbon on the rights of the patient [Internet]. 1981. Available from: www.wma.net [Accessed: May 05, 2023]

[20] Koleva I, Yoshinov B, Gerenova J, Dimitrov T, Traykovska A, Yoshinov RR. Bioethics and Physical medicine: From the heritage of Asclepius and Hippocrates to the contemporary rehabilitation clinical practice. In: Current Innovations in Medicine and Medical Science. Vol. 7. London: BPI; 2022. pp. 42-66. DOI: 10.9734/bpi/cimms/v7/8594F

[21] Blackburn E, Durocher E, Feldman D, Hudon A, Laliberté M, Mazer B, et al. Supporting, promoting, respecting and advocating: A scoping study of rehabilitation professionals' responses to patient autonomy. Canadian Journal of Bioethics. 2018;**1**:22-34. DOI: 10.7202/1058249ar

[22] Uddin T, Shakoor MA, Rathore FA, Sakel M. Ethical issues and dilemmas in spinal cord injury rehabilitation in the developing world: A mixed-method study. Spinal Cord. 2022;**5**:1-6

[23] Ghoshal A, Salins N, Damani A, Chowdhury J, Chitre A, Muckaden MA, et al. To tell or not to tell: Exploring the preferences and attitudes of patients and family caregivers on disclosure of a cancer-related diagnosis and prognosis. Journal of Global Oncology. 2019;**5**:1-12. DOI: 10.1200/JGO.19.00132

[24] Chaturvedi SK. Ethical dilemmas in palliative care in traditional developing societies, with special reference to the Indian setting. Journal of Medical Ethics. 2008;**34**(8):611-615. DOI: 10.1136/jme.2006.018887

[25] World Medical Association. WMA Declaration of Berlin on Discrimination against Elderly Individuals within Healthcare Settings [Internet]. 2022. Available from: www.wma.net [Accessed: May 05, 2023]

[26] Department of Health, Education, and Welfare. Office of the Secretary: Protection of Human Subjects. Belmont Report: Ethical principles and guidelines for the protection of human subjects of research. Report of the National Commission for the Protection of Human Subjects of Biomedical and Behavioral Research. Agency: Department of Health, Education, and Welfare. Action: Notice of Report for Public Comment. Federal Register. 1979;**44**(76):23192-23197

[27] Katz J. The Nuremberg code and the Nuremberg trial: A reappraisal. Journal of the American Medical Association. 1996;**276**(20):1662-1666. DOI: 10.1001/jama.1996.03540200048030

[28] World Medical Association. Declaration of Helsinki. Ethical principles for medical research involving human subjects [Internet]. 2013. Available from: https://www.wma.net/policies-post/wma-declaration-of-helsinki-ethical-principles-for-medical-research-involving-human-subjects/ [Accessed: March 09, 2018]

[29] World Federation for Medical Education. Global Standards for Quality Improvement: Basic Medical Education. The 2020 revision [Internet]. Available from: www.wfme.org [Accessed: May 15, 2023]

[30] Grant J. Principles of contextual curriculum design. Chapter 5. In: Swanwick T, Forrest K, O'Brien BC, editors. Understanding Medical Education. Evidence, Theory and Practice. Third ed. Oxford: Wiley Blackwell; 2019. pp. 71-88

[31] World Federation for Medical Education. Standards for distributed and distance learning in medical education [Internet]. 2021. pp. 1-48. Available from: www.wfme.org [Accessed: May 17, 2023]

[32] Koleva I, Hadjiyanev A, Yoshinov B. Electronic learning using an e-book in neurorehabilitation and neuroergotherapy for medical specialists and health professionals, members of the multi-disciplinary neurorehabilitation team. In: 14th International Technology, Education and Development Conference, Valencia, Spain, 2-4 March, 2020. INTED2020 Proceedings. Valencia: IATED; 2020. pp. 6488-6494. DOI: 10.21125/inted.2020. ISBN: 978-84-09-17939-8. ISSN: 2340-1079

[33] Koleva I, Yoshinov B, Yoshinov R. Bases of Neurorehabilitation: E-book. Sofia: SIMEL; 2020. pp. 1-584

[34] Koleva I, Yoshinov B, Yoshinov R. Rehabilitation in SARSCoV2: Structuration of an educational module and evaluation of students' competences and satisfaction. In: 14th Annual International Conference of Education, Research and Innovation. Online Conference. 8-9 November, 2021. ICERI2021 Proceedings. IATED; 2021. pp. 3266-3274. DOI: 10.21125/iceri.2021. ISBN: 978-84-09-34549-6. ISSN: 2340-1095

[35] Yoshinov R, Yoshinov B, Koleva IB. Introduction of electronic learning in the educational module "ICT-based neurorehabilitation of Neuro-COVID" with clinical cases. In: 17th International Technology, Education and Development Conference, Valencia, Spain, 6-8 March, 2023. INTED2023 Proceedings of Conference. Valencia: IATED; 2023. pp. 2158-2165. DOI: 10.21125/inted.2023. ISBN: 978-84-09-49026-4. ISSN: 2340-1079

Chapter 8

ELSI Challenges with Children in Translational Medicine

Sara Casati and Bridget Ellul

Abstract

Paediatric translational research deals mainly with genomics of biological samples. It has benefitted substantially from developments in new technologies and from international collaboration to access and use large cohorts of banked biological samples and associated data. However, there are still significant ELSI (ethical, legal and societal implications) challenges that need to be addressed before we can move smoothly from the "bench" to the "bedside" to the "community". In this chapter we shall concentrate on the intertwined ethical and legal issues regarding informed assent/consent of minors and the return of genomic results to minors and families. This leads to the societal issues faced in minor engagement and empowerment. We will then emphasise the need for healthcare integrated biobanking to maximise use of samples and data and so facilitate translational research.

Keywords: minor engagement, vulnerable research participants, informed assent - consent and dissent, tailored dialogue, return of results, healthcare integrated biobanking, responsible research & innovation – RRI, research ethics committee – REC, responsible translational research

1. Introduction

The European Society for Translational Medicine clearly defines Translational Medicine (TM) as:

"...an inter-disciplinary branch of the biomedical field supported by three main pillars: benchside, bedside and community. The goal of TM is to combine disciplines, resources, expertise, and techniques within these pillars to promote enhancements in prevention, diagnosis, and therapies" [1].

This definition inspires us because of its clear description of the two-way relationship between clinical practice and research and, more importantly, because it introduces the concept of community as a determining pillar. Translational medicine promises to improve health care for future populations by translating scientific knowledge from laboratory studies to clinical research to medical applications, including new treatments and preventive measures. This has now become a more realistic vision as scientists have access to biobanking facilities across the globe, facilitating and enhancing transnational collaboration.

Basic research on biological tissues has been boosted by the technological advances in omics, in particular genomic technology, and in bioinformatics handling big data, which promise to unravel the aetiology of rare and common diseases, with the vision of precision and prevention medicine, thus amplifying the necessity to regenerate risk assessment, ethical review, informed assent/consent and supervisory governance processes within a framework of Responsible Research and Innovation (RRI).

This evolution in medicine is critical for children opening new opportunities of children-tailored treatments in paediatric practice, which is not only characterised by a high percentage of rare diseases with a genetic aetiology but is also encumbered with a lack of medicines, specifically targeted for children [2].

Moreover, we cannot emphasise the importance of translational research on "outcomes and effectiveness in populations" [3], of crucial importance to the development of health policies for future generations. So, we prefer to talk about research with children, rather than limit ourselves to paediatric research, which primarily focuses on the clinical aspects.

In this chapter we will use the term child within the context referred to in the *Convention on the Rights of the Child* (CRC) [4], which defines a child as "every human being below the age of eighteen years unless under the law applicable to the child, majority is attained earlier". This convention has been internationally recognised, being ratified by 196 states, with the United States (US) being just a signatory [5], making it "the most widely ratified human rights treaty in the world". The rights it incorporates are a "set of universal standards or norms rooted in formal entitlement to their fulfilment and corresponding obligations on those providing that guarantee" [6].

Research with, and for, children is of special importance because it deals with a significantly higher proportion of genomic research, primarily on biological samples from children with rare diseases, but it is also available for epigenetic studies that may be predictive of risk for chronic disease in future adulthood. However, there is a major issue with the scarce availability of biological material to study, from a single country.

Moreover, this is coupled by the constraints of intertwined ethical, legal and societal issues (ELSI), primarily centred on two aspects:

> *....the ethical and legal issues of obtaining informed assent/consent for research participation by children, who are unable to provide legal consent, with ethical consideration of balancing benefits and risks to participants and to scientific progress; and.*
>
> *.....the ethical and social issues associated with the return of results that might be relevant to both the current family and to future generations, compounded by legal issues of privacy and data protection.*

Research with children offers the possibility of long-term study, throughout the transition into adulthood, and even beyond, to provide information on disease development and the effects of medical management, including therapy, over a long period of time. Engagement of child participants is crucial to ensure long-term contact with children and follow up into adult life.

Finally, it is important to consider the societal impact on translational research in children. A primary condition to ensure participation in research, particularly if provision of biological samples is required, is the infrastructure and openness of both an informational environment and a multi-actor inclusive research ecosystem. It is no coincidence that among the main assets (policy agendas) of RRI[1] [7] there are: scientific education, which is increasingly being implemented as scientific citizenship, public engagement, which soon turned into multi-actor engagement, open access and social justice and inclusion, especially to avoid unfair discrimination of particular groups in research.

Translational and Prevention Medicine progressively based on omics and big data [8] research, and healthcare integrated biobanking, can develop only through systemic community engagement, where young generations with their families become a pillar of the community. Raising awareness [9], making science practices and processes familiar, inclusion and engagement in scientific debates [10], transparency, participatory assenting/consenting, and governance are ELSI/RRI conditions to become scientific citizens and to collaborate in translational research. They are requirements for a responsible, quality practice in research [11].

2. Informed assent/consent and dissent

2.1 Assent and consent as an ethical-normative process

Since the Nuremberg Code, informed consent has been considered an essential condition to develop any research, the backbone of ethical and responsible research, as it should enforce and respect the willing, the autonomy of the potential participant guaranteeing sufficient knowledge and comprehension and a space of empowerment to exercise free power of choice and make an understanding, enlightened decision [12]. Moreover, the Code embodies what we now consider as the RRI horizon, particularly in the statement: "The duty and responsibility for ascertaining the quality of the consent rests upon each individual who initiates, directs, or engages in the experiment". This *de facto* introduced the informed consent as a process in dialogue between participant and researcher/clinician whose ethicality and consistency lie in the transparency, verifiability and accessibility of the research process that is proposed as well as in the responsible and documented verification by the research professional of the potential participant's comprehension. If this represents a practical challenge with adults, which is concretely outlined in Article 29 of the European *Clinical Trials Regulation 536/2014*, particularly in the passage reiterating that the research team must during the interview first and foremost respond to the information need of the potential participant or patient populations at stake in that research [13], with minors it implies a real paradigm shift.

From an ethical point of view, there has been an immense stepwise change in just a few years: from parental/guardian consent as a *sine qua non* for a research study, there has been a shift to positive consent of the child, a practical/ethical consent: the child is the participant, not the parents. In an ELSI horizon, this represents a significant challenge involving the child as a participant, who progressively acquires decision-making competence and legal capacity.

[1] For over 20 years, Europe, with its bodies, is clearly fostering both participatory science and innovation through the breakthrough paradigm of RRI that aims at producing science and innovation in partnership with/responding to society, being highly competitive and at the same time respectful of human rights, sustainable (economically and environmental), and transferrable.

This means profoundly rethinking assent and consent as a dynamic, step-by-step process based on an ongoing dialogue between children, parents and researchers/biobankers, from the proposal till the reuse and secondary use and data and results access and moving toward dynamic and participatory models of regulation and interpretation. Since obtaining informed assent/consent is a process that evolves over time as children develop and mature, and will most likely extend into adulthood, we would prefer to talk about assenting/consenting for research in children to emphasise the ongoing engagement between researchers and participants.

Moreover, as children grow and gain capacity, minors highlight the direct link between consent at maturity, follow-up, and engagement, which is critical to sustainable and fair/FAIR (Findable, Accessible, Interoperable, Reusable) biobanking for our future.

It has not been an obvious process, deconstructing patterns, a long journey of inclusion and recognition of the minor as a participant, whose opinion must be considered and whose dissent must be respected. At the same time, it outlines the path of making researchers and biobankers aware of their role in increasing the risk of vulnerability and discrimination of minors involved in biobank-based research, if not acted upon responsibly, inclusive and guarantor of empowerment, and capability settings.

It took 50 years to deconstruct the paternalistic paradigm, to include the minor, the most protected subject through the regulatory framework, to respect them by providing and encouraging processes and tools of self-determination, such as agreement/assent, dissent and consent at maturity. The conception of these terms and their definition has also evolved and is addressed in the next Section 2.1.1, which follows their progressive development.

It is indicative that the regulatory framework revolves primarily around clinical trials, biomedical research in a strict sense. Only in 2006 did the Council of Europe publish the first recommendation on research on biological material of human origin [14], which served as one of the first building blocks for an ELSI framework for translational medicine and research biobanking involving children. This 50-year-long responsible bioethical evolution (revolution) has been possible thanks to soft laws that promote and recommend but do not impose good practices and fairness.

2.1.1 The ELSI evolution

Children, who are still minors, that is below the legal age for consent in a particular country, have a right to give their opinion, as laid out in article 12 of the *Convention on the Rights of the Child*, which states that a mature child "capable of forming his or her own views" has "the right to express those views freely in all matters..., the views of the child being given due weight in accordance with the age and maturity of the child" [4]. This agreement by the child is known as assent, and must be accompanied by the permission of the parents or guardians, to provide valid consent, as a safeguard for ethical research [15].

However, as will be discussed below, there is wide variation across countries in the practical procedures employed to obtain assent from potential child participants and legal "consent" or permission from their parents, reflecting the differences in national law regarding who is competent to provide legally valid consent. This may be problematic for international collaborative research, including biobanking. Moreover, the *General Data Protection Regulation* (*GDPR*) has added another confounding legal requirement for European research, since explicit legal consent is one of the mechanisms that make data processing lawful in Article 6(1)(a) [16].

The *Declaration of Helsinki* introduced assent by minors in the 2000 version, as basic principle 25: "When a subject deemed legally incompetent, such as a minor child, is able to give assent to decisions about participation in research, the investigator must obtain that assent in addition to the consent of the legally authorised representative" [17].

Assent was not mentioned in the *2001 Directive on Clinical Trials*, where Article 4(a) states that the informed consent of the parents "must represent the minor's presumed will" [18] but with the subsequent Regulation, assent was recognised as a national requirement in some countries. In the 2002 Council for International Organisations of Medical Sciences (CIOMS) Guidelines, prepared in collaboration with the World Health Organisation (WHO), there is mention of "knowing agreement, sometimes referred to as assent" [19] but by the next revision in 2016 [20], assent is recognised as a process.

The role of children as research participants is now widely accepted but it was through clinical trial research that the rights of children in research were highlighted. So not surprisingly, the early definitions of assent/consent for research with children are enshrined in regulations regarding clinical trials, at least in the European Union (EU).

The EU legislation regulating Clinical Trials defines minors under Article 2, as subjects "under the age of legal competence to give informed consent" and proceeds to define informed consent for minors as "an authorisation or agreement from their legally designated representative to include them in the clinical trial" [13]. Although Article 32(2) states that "a minor shall take part in the informed consent procedure in a way adapted to his or her age and mental maturity", Article 29(8) states that assent is only mandatory for "a minor who is capable of forming an opinion and assessing the information given to him or her" only when required by national law.

Meanwhile in the US, the *Code of Federal Regulations, 45CFR 46* for the Protection of Human Subjects, Section 46.402, defines assent as "a child's affirmative agreement to participate in research. Mere failure to object should not, absent affirmative agreement, be construed as assent" and defines permission as "the agreement of parent(s) or guardian to the participation of their child or ward in research" [21].

Moreover, the EU Recommendations of the Expert Group for the implementation of the Regulation define assent as "a statement of will with legal value according to national law" but proceed to recommend that even in the absence of such legal requirement, researchers should ask for an agreement from the minor, the term agreement being used "by analogy to "assent" where it is not a legal requirement" [22]. Moreover, in many countries, Research Ethics Committees (RECs) are increasingly requiring child assent for any research project on minors [23].

In any case, the *Clinical Trials Regulation* explicitly requires children and young people to "take part" in the assent/consent process: the minor participates while the legally designated representatives authorise their participation. Under this regard, Article 32 (1c) is critical and fully recognises the minor as the participant, stating that "the explicit wish of a minor who is capable of forming an opinion and assessing the information referred to in Article 29(2) to refuse participation in, or to withdraw from, the clinical trial at any time, is respected by the investigator" [13]. The Regulation also articulates how informed assent/consent is a process configured by researchers or research team members trained or experienced in working with children and shaped based on the informational need of the person who has to understand and assent/consent. This is an RRI pillar: a research proposal and the information to "assent" can only be shared with/by competent and "responsible" personnel in dialogue with the potential participant.

The 2016 updated Recommendation by the Council of Europe, firmly in dialogue with the Oviedo Convention, and its additional protocols, highlights this change of pace in Article 12(4): "If the person not able to consent is a minor, his/her opinion should be taken into consideration as an increasingly determining factor in proportion to age and degree of maturity. Any objection by the person not able to consent should be respected. Any wishes previously expressed by such a person should be taken into account" [14].

This is echoed in the 2016 CIOMS, Guideline 17, which states that children 'who are too immature to give assent" may still communicate a "deliberate objection", that is "an expression of disapproval or refusal of a proposed procedure". The Regulation regarding Clinical Trials in Article 32.1(c) refers to an objection by children who have the capacity to take decisions, which implies that dissent is the "lack of assent". The expert group states that dissent is "the expression of the minor's will to refuse participation in a trial" and that where assent is required by national law, dissent is equated with a definite refusal to participate in a trial. The researcher should be aware that dissent may be expressed in writing or orally but also by non-verbal means of communication.

Also, consent must be obtained at the legal age of consent, to allow a clinical trial to continue into adulthood. Article 32.3 of the *Clinical Trials Regulation* emphasises that the "express informed consent shall be obtained before that subject can continue to participate in the clinical trial" [13]. Similarly Article 12 (5) of *Rec (2016)6* states that "Where a person not able to consent, whose biological materials have been stored for future research, attains or regains the capacity to consent, reasonable efforts should be made to seek the consent of that person for continued storage and research use of his or her biological materials" [14].

In ELSI words, the consent of the young person attaining the legal age is needed for continued biobanking, and this consent is *de facto* the first full consent expressed after the long assenting process built on the child's assent as well as parents/guardians' permission to biobank.

In the last few years, this change based on the inclusion and engagement of children has become pervasive. The CIOMS together with WHO suggest not only that "Children and adolescents must be included in health-related research unless a good scientific reason justifies their exclusion..." [20] in full agreement with both the RRI [24] asset of Social Justice & Inclusion which avoids unfair exclusion of particular groups from either participation in research and/or access to benefits arising from research, and the Council of Europe's current challenge to improve participation of children in the decision-making process on matters regarding their health [25].

Moreover, these international, global ethical guidelines for Health-related Research Involving Humans underline that before undertaking research involving children and adolescents, the researcher and the REC (and we add the biobanks/biobankers too) must ensure that: "the agreement (assent) of the child or adolescent has been obtained in keeping with the child's or adolescent's capacity, after having been provided with adequate information about the research tailored to the child's or adolescent's level of maturity" [20].

In fact, to give assent the child or adolescent is meaningfully engaged in the research discussion in accordance with their capacities. And as CIOMS guidelines underline "The process of obtaining assent must take into account not only the age of children, but also their individual circumstances, life experiences, emotional and psychological maturity, intellectual capabilities and the child's or adolescent's family situation" [20]. Such circumstances can play a key role in determining the child's risk of vulnerability.

Finally, the CIOMS Guidelines stress that adolescents who reach the legal age of consent during the study are to decide if they want to continue participation or not and this decision overrides that previously given by their parents [20].

2.1.2 The child as a vulnerable in transition in research

Children are "...entitled to special care and assistance" [26] and "shall have the right to such protection and care as is necessary for their well-being" [27] because of both a risk of conditioning, due to the differential power relationships between adults (researchers, parents, guardians) and child participants, and a risk of manipulation in interaction with adults. They can be particularly exposed to an increased risk of vulnerability by:

- potential discrimination (exclusion of children with disabilities, refugees, orphans...);

- overprotection (without research specific to minors, they would suffer from the lack of development of tailored diagnosis and treatments).

But a child is a person in evolution with a vulnerability in a transition. Their vulnerability does not arise from disorders or predisposition, except in specific cases. It is a temporary vulnerability that can be increased if the adult ecosystem (researchers, parents, guardians, etc.) does not recognise children as human beings to be respected, and listened to, and valued. The participation of young people in all aspects of their personal and social development is a fundamental right; the ELSI challenge is to guarantee and provide capability/empowerment settings and inclusive environments to equip children, but also adults, to ensure children's participation in the healthcare and research knowledge and decision making. Thus, children are counter intuitively special: they are temporarily vulnerable persons, being in a process of accelerated evolution and ethically requesting empowerment and respect for their full human development.

Biobanking with children and their engagement in TM should prove an ideal training ground for both RRI and scientific citizenship, fostering the cultural change for collaborative and participatory science. Their involvement implies the need to tackle inescapable ELSI issues that if not addressed increase vulnerability in all individuals at risk, not just children, as well as imply an irresponsibility, an unprofessionalism of the researcher, of the biobanker.

After the Nazi experiments, which exposed the human beings involved and used them as guinea pigs to the absolute vulnerability, the Nuremberg Code establishes a point of no return by recognising the free and informed consent of the potential participant as a prerequisite for research.

Here begins a long journey of inclusion and recognition of the other as a participant, still in progress, and of making researchers aware of their own role, in increasing the risk of vulnerability of individuals involved in the research, if not acted upon responsibly.

In 1974, the National Commission for the Protection of Human Subjects of Biomedical and Behavioural Research highlighted that "Respect for persons incorporates at least two ethical convictions: i. first, that individuals should be treated as autonomous agents, ii. and second, that persons with diminished autonomy are entitled to protection. The principle of respect for persons thus divides into two separate moral requirements: the requirement to acknowledge autonomy and the requirement to protect those with diminished autonomy" [28].

However, the Belmont Report declines respect for persons not yet capable of full autonomy, for instance for minors, beyond mere protection, envisaging to give them the opportunity to choose what shall or shall not happen to them, and whether, or not, to participate in research to the degree that they are capable.

The Report introduces a key concept in terms of RRI and participatory biobanking with both children and vulnerables, highlighting that to respect persons one must give consideration and substantial weight to all the actors at stake, including the potential participants, balancing their right to be especially protected and at the same time empowered and enabled to participate in research.

The Report is also a pioneer in introducing the role of third parties to acknowledge vulnerables' wishes and to protect them from harm. RECs as well as biobanks can be considered as the third party for excellence within the research biobanking and TM horizon: as shared before, their role in recognising and including minors as participants, as well as guaranteeing their rights and promoting their capabilities, is central.

Twenty years later the Barcelona Declaration [29] strengthens this RRI principle balancing protection and capacity-building guarantee. In fact, the care, and the protection for the vulnerable, for those whose autonomy or dignity or integrity are capable of being threatened, are core principles. But the principle also specifically requires not merely non-interference with the autonomy, dignity or integrity of beings, but also that they receive assistance to enable them to realise their potential.

Subsequent research ethics guidelines follow The Belmont Report in linking vulnerability to consent, exploitation and special protections. For example, the *Declaration on Bioethics and Human Rights* stipulated in Article 8 that "In applying and advancing scientific knowledge, medical practice and associated technologies, human vulnerability should be taken into account. Individuals and groups of special vulnerability should be protected, and the personal integrity of such individuals respected" [30].

Meanwhile, CIOMS in its Guideline 15 invokes "special protections" and reaffirms the role of third parties: "When vulnerable individuals and groups are considered for recruitment in research, researchers and research ethics committees must ensure that specific protections are in place to safeguard the rights and welfare of these individuals and groups in the conduct of the research" [31]. They should "promote voluntary decision-making, limit the potential for confidentiality breaches, and ...protect the interests" of the vulnerable [31]. Recommended safeguards include the request for an intermediary to obtain assent/consent, the use of consent materials appropriate for the participant and adequate data protection measures, such as pseudonymisation and secure data storage systems.

The notion of universal vulnerability (fragility or susceptibility to suffering, linked to human embodiment) underpins ethical concern for all research participants. But universal vulnerability is not explicitly identified in research ethics guidelines. Instead, there is an assumed "normal" research participant for whom standard ethical protections are adequate. This baseline normal research participant is characterised by Luna as "mature, moderately well-educated, clear thinking, literate, [and] self-supporting" [32]. Vulnerable participants are identified against this implicit norm and their vulnerability is essentially specific and relational: they are vulnerable to agents regarding particular threats, and individuals are vulnerable because they are especially susceptible to harm or exploitation by others. Only 3 Guidelines define special vulnerability from CIOMS [31], Canadian Tri-Council [33] and International Conference on Harmonisation (ICH), in its glossary [34].

CIOMS and the Canadian Tri-Council Policy Statement define vulnerability in terms of decreased ability to protect one's own interests, secondary to intra-personal factors (e.g., reduced capacity to give informed consent) or contextual factors (e.g., limited access to social goods including rights, opportunities and power).

RECs and biobanks are charged with ensuring that additional safeguards to protect the rights and welfare of subjects who are likely to be vulnerable are included (directly or just by providing their samples and data) in the research under review. To make this determination, they might be advised to consider questions such as: (1) is inclusion necessary? and (2) if so, are safeguards adequate?

In parallel, they play, together with the Research Infrastructures, a central role within the research ecosystem to empower and engage children and families as well as researchers and clinicians as a team, to support an inclusive scientific community based on transparency, inclusion, mutual recognition and openness. Biobanking and TM with children grow and we need an ethically healthy balance between the protection of vulnerable persons, a risk/mitigation assessment competence, and the development of a fair/FAIR research in the age of omics medicine: it is critical to support researchers/clinicians in rethinking the assenting/consenting process with minors to fully recognise and include them, stepping forward the risk of vulnerability via participation.

2.2 Not just information but tailored dialogue

2.2.1 Comprehension and informational tools

Full informed consent from adult research participants can only be provided when they have "competence or decisional capacity... to understand material information, appreciate the situation and its consequences... and communicate a choice" [35]. The same requirements can and should be considered for capacity to provide informed assent.

According to McGregor and Ott [36], capacity to consent can be considered as having four elements: "(1) understanding the information relevant to make a decision, (2) appreciating how the decision will impact them personally, (3) manipulating the information rationally and reasoning, and (4) communicating a voluntary choice".

For research with children, information is provided not only to the legally designated representatives but also to the minor, when it must be "tailored to the child's or adolescent's level of maturity" [20] or as the *Clinical Trials Regulation*, Article 32(1)(b) requires, "adapted to their age and mental maturity" [13]. However, "age only partly correlates with maturity" [22]. Increased maturity is related to age since the skills to understand the information provided develop as the child grows, but more importantly competence depends on mental development, with cognitive capabilities and decisional capacity increasing and evolving with age. In the US, Institutional Review Boards (IRBs) are empowered to ascertain if "children are capable of assenting" by considering the ages, maturity, and psychological state of the children involved" [21].

Since maturity is also related to socio-economic factors, such as "educational level and belief system" [37], health status, culture and family dynamics [38], using age as an indicator for capacity to assent is not sufficient. But using age groups to produce guidelines for procedures to engage child participants acts as "a practical instrument" [22].

Various studies have tried to determine the level of understanding at different ages, so as to establish an age of assent, but there is no agreed decision. The American Academy of Paediatrics and the National Commission for the Protection of Human Subjects of Biomedical and Behavioural Research recommend assent for children above 7 years of age [39]. It is generally agreed that adolescents are competent to make decisions regarding research participation. However even here the age groups used vary markedly from 10 to 19 years by WHO [40] to 10–18 years by the Expert Group on Clinical trials [21] to 11–21-year-olds by the American Academy of Paediatrics [41].

Hein argues that children aged 12 and above are able to provide informed consent rather than assent [42]. This is based on her previous studies using the modified MacArthur Competence Assessment Tool for Clinical Research (MacCAT-CR) to assess children's decision-making capacity, where it was established that children aged 11.2 years and above were competent to agree to research participation while those below 9.6 years were not, with those in between being 'in transition' with increasing capacities [43].

However, in the EU, there is no agreement on specified ages for consent and assent in research with children, as evidenced by the survey led by the Working Group on Ethics at the European Network of Paediatric Research at the European Medicines Agency (EnprEMA) [44], with age for assent starting at 4 years old, while the legal age for informed consent varies between 14 and 18 years [45].

Even legal maturity is arbitrarily assigned a specific age by a country or by individual states in the US, generally the age of 18 years. In the States, this has led to the legal recognition of "emancipated" or "mature" minors who are legally allowed to provide informed consent without the need for their parents' consent, or even without the parents' awareness about their involvement in research. Minors who are married or join the US Armed Forces obtain automatic emancipation. In some US states, other minors, such as those who are pregnant, or parents themselves or living independently, can be emancipated through a declaration by the Courts. In the United Kingdom [46], children over 16 are legally able to give consent for participation in clinical trials but there is no legal statute governing other types of research. Some have therefore argued that Gillick competence should also apply [47].

Finally, there are no specific guidelines as to how the researcher should ensure that the potential participant has really understood the information provided. Although Article 31(1)b of the *Clinical Trials Regulation* requires the potential child participant to be provided with information that is "adequate in view of their capacity to understand it", it does not make comprehension mandatory for the child as required for the parent by Article 29(5), which states that "it shall be verified that the subject has understood the information" [13].

The Recommendations of the Expert Group on Clinical Trials with children recommend that the information provided should be ethically approved and the material provided to children checked "for sufficient understanding in the relevant" group of children, but there is no specific guideline for the research team.

Researchers are now developing tools to check understanding, such as the modified Quality of Informed Consent [48, 49]. A recent review [50] only identified 19 studies that used tools to assess comprehension of children during the assenting process, of which only seven studies were from real research studies. The tools used were mainly questionnaires with either multiple choice questions or open-ended questions but there were also interviews and observations. The review did suggest that the use of "enhanced paper forms (e.g., by simplified text or illustrations)" was useful. The paucity of the literature underlies the importance of research on this topic and the need to develop assent models for children.

Children as potential participants must be provided with relevant information that allows a free decision about participation in a proposed study. This should include information about the aims, methods, benefits and risks of the study, as well as details related to the rights of the participant, such as the right to withdraw from research at any time and the right to confidentiality. Children's concerns may be different from those of their parents [51], so the information has to be tailored to their needs, which will become more obvious depending on how strong an engagement there is between the research team and the children/adolescents. However, the information should be targeted to the capacity of the child [52] and be in "a language or another form of communication that the individual can understand" [53].

Another practical aspect that determines understanding is how the information is communicated. The *Clinical Trials Regulation*, Article 32(1)(b) states that only "investigators or members of the investigating team who are trained or experienced in working with children" [13] should provide information. The researcher should use patience and sensitivity in communication [37] and provide sufficient time to be asked questions to clarify any issues, maybe alone rather than in the presence of parents. The research team must remain aware of the family dynamics, which may indirectly affect the child's decision to participate or not.

One has to consider the amount of information provided as well as the type of material used for facilitating comprehension. Article 29(4) of the *Clinical Trials Regulation* recommends "special attention shall be paid to the information needs of specific patient populations and of individual subjects, as well as to the methods used to give the information" [13]. The Expert Recommendations for Clinical Trials recommend that initially there should be provision of two separate sheets "one with a summary, and the other with more detailed information" [22] [to both children and their parents, so as not to overload them. Detailed information is to be provided only once they show an interest in learning more. This is good practice for a dynamic and tailored assenting process that evolves over time.

2.3 The role of research ethics committees

Research Ethics Committees (RECs), because of their third-party role, guarantee special protection and empowerment for children participating in research as highlighted in the section on vulnerability. They provide an independent review of the research proposal, ensuring that not only are ethical principles being addressed but there is definite feasibility of the outlined procedures being fulfilled by the research team. This provides an additional safeguard for responsible translational research with children, in particular with regard to ensuring informed assent from children below the legal age of consent. Ideally RECs should ensure that the children and parents were involved in the study design [54]. RECs evaluate and can require modifications to the proposed format of information being provided, methodology applied during the dialogue with participants and the tools supporting the assenting process such as information Sheets and Assent forms [55].

RECs are an important safeguard for clinical research where the clinician is the researcher, as they generally require intermediaries to communicate with potential participants and obtain their assent/consent. This is particularly important when the clinician is also the principal investigator and who may therefore be the cause of therapeutic misconception and/or who may have a conflict of interest in relation to research funding.

In addition, under special circumstances (like during the Covid epidemic) RECs are able to consider waivers of consent and assent when it would otherwise be impractical to carry out the research, which is deemed to be of minimal risk and of significant social benefit [54]. In practice, RECs may waive parental consent if it is considered to be detrimental to the child [56], due to conflict between the children and their parents, or even harm by the parents, for example, for research on drug use, domestic abuse, child abuse and reproductive and sexuality issues [20].

In the US, recommendations to introduce assent and involve IRBs were introduced in the late 1970s [57] and there is federal legislation [21] requiring assent from children (below the legal age for consent) participating in research and permission from the parent(s) or guardian, unless assent is waived by an IRB [21]. IRBs also are empowered to waive parental permission in such cases [1]. Furthermore, a waiver to child assent can be applied by IRBs if the children are deemed to be of such limited capacity to assent that they cannot be engaged in decision making, or if the proposed research is of absolute benefit to that group of children and can only be obtained through that specific research even if there is greater than minimal risk [21]. In cases of waiver, the IRB will require further protection of the child, e.g., by appointing an advocate or guardian to accompany the child in the research process. The IRB can also authorise waivers for parental permission for emancipated minors, who are able to provide legal consent.

3. Return of results

Technological developments in genomic research with the production of large amounts of data and the exploratory analysis of gene variants, mirroring the trend in healthcare, have led to a growing problem with respect to an increased potential for findings unrelated to the aims of the study. These can be incidental findings that are totally unexpected or less commonly secondary findings that are actively searched for during the study but unrelated to the research aims. So current literature is discussing individual research results to include all types of results. What is uniformly accepted is that all research results have to be validated [58, 59] by confirming the result in an accredited laboratory before being returned.

It is always recommended to discuss and decide on return (or not) of results at the time of dialogue in the assenting/consenting process [60]. Dynamic consent would allow participants to change their preferences.

Moreover, in the translational context [61], with the new omics technology [62], it has become crucial to consider the effect all results would have on the participants, right from the start of developing the study protocol. Genomic counsellors should be part of the research team to evaluate risks versus benefits to participants during the study and to offer their services beyond the study, to the participant's when their healthcare is affected and extended family if appropriate.

3.1 Which result?

In Europe, the *Additional Protocol to the Convention on Human Rights and Biomedicine* is clear that results relevant to the "current or future health or quality of life of research participants" must be offered together with "health care or counselling" [63], reiterated also in *Rec (2016)6* [14]. Although in the United States there is no federal law mandating return of research results, changes to the Common Rule in 2017 [64] require researchers to inform participants during the consent process whether "clinically relevant research results, including individual research results" will be returned [65].

It is now generally accepted that research participants should receive all research results [65], including genomic research results [66–68] not just if these are of benefit to the participant. The public, patients and participants support and want to receive results [65], although research also shows that the more knowledge made available to the participant, including counselling, the less strong was the desire for results [68–71]. On the other hand, the scientific and health professionals are more restrained about disclosing information [68, 70], mirroring the ethical and legal challenges related to disclosure. This is even more relevant in research with children because it is often genomic research and moreover children have a long future ahead, so any possible healthcare intervention should be as early as possible.

So, any results that warrant an action should be returned. "Actionable" has been defined as follows: "if there are available preventive and/or treatment measures and the disorder has either (i) childhood onset and such measures are therefore initiated in childhood, or (ii) adult onset, but such measures have been demonstrated to be effective when started in childhood" [72]. As of 2021, the Clinical Genome Resource Paediatric Actionability Working Group was able to provide guidelines regarding return of results related to 143 genes, on the basis of actionability [73].

The American College of Medical Genetics and Genomics (ACMG) guidelines to assist in return of secondary findings following clinical gene sequencing [74] recommend not to return results related to adult-onset non-treatable disease but to report findings related to adult-onset conditions that are treatable only in adult life, because of potential benefit to the parents or other family members [75], also labelled as "personal utility" to the health or reproductive decisions of the relatives [76].

These ACMG guidelines have been used to develop guidelines for research practice. A particular set of guidelines that concentrate on the preferences of children and their parents [76] decided that results for adult-onset diseases, non-treatable diseases and carrier status would not be disclosed to children below 18 years; adolescents in these guidelines are 13–17-year-olds.

3.2 To whom?

Parents believe they have a right to be given results from genomic research on their children [71, 77] even for results unrelated to the main aims of the study [58] and also irrespective of actionability [78]. However, this practice threatens the child's right to an "open future", that is the parents receiving all the information can undermine the right of the children to decide for themselves in future.

Research participants may opt not to receive results, and this should be certainly respected for mature adults [79] to respect their "right not to know" information about their health [14, 63] but if parents opt not to receive their children's actionable results, it may be necessary to obtain an ethical opinion. The European Society of Human Genetics (ESHG) and EuroGentest recommend that the final decision on return of serious and actionable incidental findings should be made by professionals [59]. The researcher may have a duty to override the parents' right not to know [80].

Ideally parents should share the results with their children, according to their age and maturity. Adolescents should be involved together with their parents in deciding what results they want to receive [81]. Adolescents do take different independent decisions from their parents and may want less information than their parents [81]. In the case of disagreement between parents and participating children, there should be return of results if immediate action is necessary, with such decision being taken by a multidisciplinary team of geneticists, ethicists and counsellors [76].

For adult-onset disorders actionable only in adulthood, results should not be disclosed to safeguard the child's autonomy and right to decide on disclosure once they attain the legal age of consent. This view has also been supported by the public [71]. However, for genomic results, the likelihood is that the result is important for the family, including the parents, in which case benefit to the parents will also be of benefit to the child [80].

Generally, parents are prepared to share genetic results with extended family [58] but they should respect the child's autonomy by considering their preferences and assess possible risks to privacy by sharing the information; this should be balanced with the potential benefit to relatives [82]. It may be necessary to involve an ethics committee to assist in this decision, to ensure the confidentiality of genomic information is protected. They should consider this issue at the time of writing the research protocol.

Genomic technologies are used for diagnosing genetic disorders and for research, but it can be difficult to distinguish between the two [59] though it is clearly reasonable to do so [68]. However translational research encompasses both aspects and therefore, the distinction may not be necessary and guidelines for clinical care could reasonably be applied also to research.

4. Data protection issues

With the introduction of the *GDPR*, consent has taken on a legal connotation since consent is one of the mechanisms in Article 6(1)(a) that make data processing lawful [16]. Article 4(1)(11) states that this legal consent should be "freely given, specific, informed and unambiguous indication of the data subject's ... agreement to the processing of personal data concerning him or her" [16] and according to Article 9(2)(a) it should be explicit for sensitive data. However, this has to be understood as separate from the ethical need for informed assent/consent.

As mentioned by the European Data Protection Supervisor, there is "clear overlap between informed consent of human participants in research projects involving humans and consent under data protection law" [83]. Should another legal basis be applied for data protection, informed assent/consent "could still serve as an 'appropriate safeguard' of the rights of the data subject' [83].

Recital 161 of the *GDPR* states that for participation in clinical trials, the provisions of the *Clinical Trials Regulation* [13] apply, implying the age of consent to personal data processing is the same age as the age to consent for trial participation [45].

Article 8 of the *GDPR* introduces age limits for the child's consent to data processing, but only in relation to information society services. This is set at 16 years, below which parental legal consent is required, unless the state opts for a lower age, but with a minimum of 13 years. However, it appears that this has not been generally used as a guideline for setting legally valid consent for data processing in research. In particular, for clinical trial research in Europe, the legal age for consent is known to vary between 14 and 18 years [45], with the proviso that children below that age are also, as regulated by Article 32(2), involved in the informed consent procedure, thus in the assenting procedure, "in a way adapted to his or her age and mental maturity" [13].

The *GDPR* does not mention scientific research with minors, although Article 12 requires that information provided to children is in a "concise, transparent, intelligible and easily accessible form, using clear and plain language, in particular for any information addressed specifically to a child" and Recital 38 highlights the need for "specific protection" of children's "personal data, as they may be less aware of the risks, consequences and safeguards concerned and their rights in relation to the processing of personal data".

The *GDPR* also safeguards the right to withdraw consent to data processing, implying withdrawal as a research participant, at any time without suffering any repercussions. Children also have a right to withdraw their assent at any time.

Although the right to access to data processed in scientific research may be waived through derogations under Article 89(2) if "such rights are likely to render impossible or seriously impair the achievement of the specific purposes" [16], this may lead to different practices in European member states, thus complicating multinational research collaboration.

5. Healthcare integrated biobanking and engagement

Since rare diseases affect only a few individuals in a population, and most rare conditions are paediatric in onset, the rare disease community has been pioneering to ensure paediatric transnational and international collaboration to obtain large cohorts to study and to create *ante litteram* a constant translational dialogue between clinics, research and Patient/Parent Associations [84] through research biobanks and registries.

Currently it is widely recognised as a crucial requirement for Precision and Prevention Medicine to have the availability of an extensive collection of human samples (both diseased and healthy) with well-documented phenotypic data [85]. Getting timely diagnoses and treatments requires the identification of biomarkers that would be useful for early detection, prevention and treatment of diseases associated with specific medical conditions such as cancer, cardiovascular disease and many other disorders. The ability to determine specific biomarkers for disease diagnosis and prognosis of therapeutic response will have a meaningful impact on healthcare for everybody.

The European challenge to infrastructure research to support and increase collaborative, responsible quality research, has been central to infrastructure biobanking thanks to the dedicated Biobanking & Biomolecular Resources Research Infrastructure – BBMRI-ERIC [86] and its inclusive community of practices. The BBMRI-ERIC Directory, for instance, provides an aggregated overview of global biobanks and collections of samples and data that are available for research.

Omics, artificial intelligence-driven process automation, data analytics, robotics and other emerging technological advances are driving the revolution of biospecimen science, both providing new insights into the genetic component of human disease and developing an automated and more personalised approach to healthcare. This means a paradigm moving toward dynamic and participatory models of regulation, governance and interpretation within an RRI horizon as well as a translational, healthcare integrated evolution of biobanking with a direct impact for any citizen, regardless of disease or health condition.

Translational, healthcare integrated biobanking, like TM, requires the construction of a conscious community, an extended scientific community, which proactively recognises and includes as partners both the patient-citizen and the clinician, and fully regenerates and concretises research as a responsible process, precisely because it is participatory.

In conclusion: I can only be accountable for an act, for a process (be responsible for it) if I understand it, I'm conscious and both trained and engaged; just as I act responsibly for a process because I am understood by it, I am recognised as a part of it, a partner in it. As shared by the participatory community of the Italian National Node (BBMRI.it): "To contribute to, and to participate in, the biobanking process, and to take advantage of results, it is essential to be informed, and aware of the scientific process that arises from biobanking, and to understand how this innovative scientific model is set up; an innovative model, above all, because it defines personalised diagnoses and treatments and requires a re-thinking of rights, responsibilities, and choices" [87].

From proactive participation of citizenship to state-of-the-art infrastructure and global standards, to necessary regulatory controls, various issues need to be overcome to benefit from the revolutionary potential of biobanking. Patients-citizens, clinicians, researchers, and institutions altogether should rethink and regenerate the clinical practice in a horizon of scientific development through systematic, extensive data and sample collection, based on compliance with the correct (ELSI, qualitative, "institutional-organisational") and congruous requirements for potential research use.

Translational biobanking is ethical, sustainable and fair as a collaborative process and a participatory pact between all the players involved. This participatory pact represents a pact of responsibility between all the various actors involved. Giving custody and taking care of samples (being custodians and responsible for the care, but not being the owners) is the cornerstone of this participatory process. The biobank as a third party, a custodian, ensures patient/participant's participation, rights and data security, guaranteeing samples and data use and distribution consistent with the assent/consent expressed, transparent procedures, participatory governance and returning of results.

Ideally paediatric biobanks should be an integral part of healthcare services for children. This is not the prevalent scenario, except for certain countries, such as Italy [88]. This situation maximises collection and use of biological material, which is important for any childhood condition. There should also be population-based biobanks with a paediatric focus, to collect biospecimens from unselected healthy children, to study genetic variants and their interaction with the socio-economic environment in health and disease, which can lead to disease prevention measures to maintain a healthy population.

6. Vision for the future

Research with children is most fruitful when there is sustained interaction with the child, supporting them throughout the entire research. This is real engagement, encompassing much more than provision of information, answering research queries and obtaining assent. It is the basis for dynamic assent and will hopefully lead to research involvement throughout adulthood. On a basic level engagement shows respect for the developing maturity of the child and increases confidence in decision making and so empowers the child. Furthermore, engagement with family is crucial to joint decision making with child participants and their parents/guardians and creates ongoing dialogue and being part of the team with researchers and clinicians in scientific development.

The advances in genomic technology and bioinformatics have opened up the field of translational research with children, now facilitated by access to substantial numbers of biological samples from children, stored in a number of worldwide paediatric biobanks, together with associated clinical data. This allows studies to be conducted on diseases that affect children, but also offers an opening to the future co-created healthcare and science horizon and practice.

Healthcare integrated biobanking, omics based and AI/machine learning-supported big data research, are core in Translational and Prevention Medicine and one of the new forms of research that impacts everyone. The younger generations, both as future citizens and as potential scientists, are at the forefront of the development, sustainability, and equity of sample-based and data-driven science, of TM. Children can eventually be paediatric patients or "next generation" patients; they may be asked to give their blood, saliva or tissues for research, as well as benefit from TM in the future. Furthermore, children are also potential "next generation" scientists, researchers and healthcare professionals. This is the world that concerns them first and foremost; the RRI shift is for them and with them.

However, multiple ELSI challenges remain. The ethical issues of obtaining informed assent highlight the need to improve the assent process, to provide adequate informational tools and to have clear policies about shared decision-making with the family. This will only be possible if we take into consideration the views of the children and their families/guardians and recognise them as partners of the research ecosystem.

It is worth mentioning the need to carry out more research on the views of adolescents and their parents to participate in research and to return of individual research results. A recent review of laws and policies regulating return of results identified the differences between 20 countries, thus proving not only a great problem to a harmonised policy but also a deterrent to international collaboration [89]. This mirrors similar discrepancies in interpretation and implementation of the same law, as is happening in Europe with the *GDPR*, where some countries are opting to introduce national derogations for scientific research, which again differ from country to country.

Nevertheless, sample-and-data-based translational research can be envisioned as a living lab, to empower children to be conscious of their scientific rights (to science, to enjoy the benefits, to participate in the scientific progress...), to take part proactively in research processes and make informed decisions about their own health. Moreover, providing children with opportunities to engage in science and become familiar with health and life science topics, handing on biobanking, can also help bridge the gap between the scientific, expert community, families and citizenship. Our aspiration is to empower and train the adult research ecosystem to include children and to recognise them as the participants while engaging and empowering the next generation in Responsible Research and Innovation.

Acknowledgements

The authors are members of the BBMRI-ERIC ELSI experts' network that brings together experts on ethical, legal and societal implications from across the National Nodes.

Dr. Sara Casati is part of the ELSI Services and Research Unit of BBMRI-ERIC as a bioethicist. This article was conceived with her BBMRI-ERIC affiliation.

Dr. Bridget Ellul, from the University of Malta, is an ELSI adviser to DwarnaBio, the national biobank in Malta and is a National Node expert from BBMRI.mt, the Malta node.

The open access fees are covered by BBMRI-ERIC.

Conflict of interest

The authors declare no conflict of interest.

BBMRI-ERIC disclaimer: Where authors are identified as personnel of the Biobanking and BioMolecular resources Research Infrastructure-European Research Infrastructure Consortium (BBMRI-ERIC), the authors alone are responsible for the views expressed in this article and they do not necessarily represent the decisions, policy or views of BBMRI-ERIC.

Notes/thanks/other declarations

This article is not the product of a specific project, rather it was inspired by several collegial exchanges over the years. Dr. Sara Casati thanks especially the BBMRI ERIC Stakeholder Forum Patient and Citizen Pillar and the CY-Biobank team for inspiration and open dialogue during various professional encounters. She also thanks colleagues and friends participating at the Paediatric Stage: Paediatric Biobanking and Minor Engagement at the EBW22 Roadshow in Rome, October 2022.

The authors also thank Michaela Th. Mayrhofer for reviewing and commenting on this proposal.

Author details

Sara Casati[1]* and Bridget Ellul[2]

1 ELSI Services and Research Unit, BBMRI-ERIC, Graz, Austria

2 University of Malta, Msida, Malta

*Address all correspondence to: sara.casati@bbmri-eric.eu

References

[1] Cohrs RJ, Martin T, Ghahramani P, Bidaut L, Higgins SA. Translational medicine definition by the European society for translational medicine. New Horizons in Translational Medicine. 2015;**2**(3):86-88. DOI: 10.1016/j.nhtm.2014.12.002

[2] EPTRI Manifesto. Available from: https://eptri.eu/wp-content/uploads/2023/03/EPTRI-MANIFESTO.pdf [Accessed: June 2, 2023]

[3] Fort DG, Herr TM, Shaw PL, Gutzman KE, Starren JB. Mapping the evolving definitions of translational research. Journal of Clinical and Translational Science. 2017;**1**(1):60-66. DOI: 10.1017/cts.2016.10. Epub 2017 Feb 2

[4] United Nations. Convention on the Rights of the Child, Adopted and Opened for Signature, RatiFication and Accession by General Assembly Resolution 44/25 of 20 November 1989, Entry into Force 2 September 1990, in Accordance with Art 49. New York, USA: United Nations; 1989. Available from: https://www.ohchr.org/en/instruments-mechanisms/instruments/convention-rights-child; [Accessed: June 2, 2023]

[5] United Nations. Geneva, Switzerland: Office of the High Commissioner of Human Rights (OHCHR); 1996-2014. Available from: https://indicators.ohchr.org/ [Accessed: June 2, 2023]

[6] Vaghri Z, Zermatten J, Lansdown G, Ruggiero R. Monitoring State Compliance with the UN Convention on the Rights of the Child. An Analysis of Attributes. Switzerland AG: Springer Nature Cham; 2022. DOI: 10.1007/978-3-030-84647-3

[7] European Commission. Directorate-General for Research and Innovation. Indicators for Promoting and Monitoring Responsible Research and Innovation – Report from the Expert Group on Policy Indicators for Responsible Research and Innovation. Luxembourg: Publications Office of the European Union; 2015. Available from: https://op.europa.eu/en/publication-detail/-/publication/306a7ab4-f3cb-46cb-b675-9697caf5df19/language-en [Accessed: January 22, 2024]

[8] Ferretti A, Ienca M, Sheehan M, et al. Ethics review of big data research: What should stay and what should be reformed? BMC Medical Ethics. 2021;**22**:51

[9] Gaskell G, Gottweis H. Biobanks need publicity. Nature. 2011;**471**:159-160. DOI: 10.1038/471159a

[10] Why researchers should resolve to engage in 2017. Nature. 2017;**541**:5. DOI: 10.1038/541005a

[11] Pain E. To be a responsible researcher, reach out and listen. Science Careers. 2017. DOI: 10.1126/science.caredit. a1700006. Available from: https://www.science.org/content/article/be-responsible-researcher-reach-out-and-listen [Accessed: January 22, 2024]

[12] Nuremberg Code. Point 1. 1947. Available from: https://research.unc.edu/human-research-ethics/resources/ccm3_019064/ [Accessed: May 16, 2023]

[13] European Union. Regulation (EU) No 536/2014 of the European Parliament and of the Council of 16 April 2014 on Clinical Trials on Medicinal Products for Human Use, and Repealing Directive 2001/20/EC., OJ L 158, 27.5. Luxembourg:

Publications Office of the European Union; 2014. pp. 1-76

[14] Council of Europe. Recommendation CM/rec(2016)6 of the Committee of Ministers to Member States on Research on Biological Materials of Human Origin. Strasbourg: Council of Europe; 2016, Available from: https://search.coe.int/cm/Pages/result_details.aspx?ObjectId=090000168064e900 [Accessed: June 15, 2023]

[15] Roth-Cline M, Nelson RM. Parental permission and child assent in research on children. The Yale Journal of Biology and Medicine. 2013;**86**(3):291-301

[16] European Union. Regulation (EU) 2016/679 of the European Parliament and of the Council of 27 April 2016 on the Protection of Natural Persons with Regard to the Processing of Personal Data and on the Free Movement of Such Data and Repealing Directive 95/46/EC (General Data Protection Regulation). OJL 119. Luxembourg: Publications Office of the European Union; 2016. pp. 1-88

[17] World Medical Association, WMA. Declaration of Helsinki – Ethical Principles for Medical Research Involving Human Subjects. Edinburgh: WMA; 2000

[18] European Union. Directive 2001/20/EC of the European Parliament and of the Council of 4 April 2001 on the Approximation of the Laws, Regulations and Administrative Provisions of the Member States Relating to the Implementation of Good Clinical Practice in the Conduct of Clinical Trials on Medicinal Products for Human Use. OJL 121. Luxembourg: Publications Office of the European Union; 2001. p. 34

[19] Council for International Organizations of Medical Sciences (CIOMS). Guideline 14. In: International Ethical Guidelines for Biomedical Research Involving Human Subjects. Geneva: CIOMS; 2002. pp. 55-56

[20] Council for International Organizations of Medical Sciences (CIOMS). Guidelines 17. In: International Ethical Guidelines for Health-Related Research Involving Humans. Geneva: CIOMS; 2016. pp. 64-68

[21] US. Code of Federal Regulations. 45 CFR 46 Protection of Human Subjects. Subpart D—Additional Protections for Children Involved as Subjects in Research. Code of Federal Regulations. Washington DC, USA: US Government Publishing Office; 1983. Available from: https://www.ecfr.gov/current/title-45/subtitle-A/subchapter-A/part-46/subpart-D?toc=1 [Accessed: June 12, 2023]

[22] European Commission. Ethical Considerations for Clinical Trials on Medicinal Products Conducted with Minors. Recommendations of the Expert Group on Clinical Trials for the Implementation of Regulation (EU) No 536/2014 on Clinical Trials on Medicinal Products for Human Use. European Commission; 2017. pp. 1-48. Available from: chrome-extension://efaidnbmnnnibpcajpcglclefindmkaj/https://health.ec.europa.eu/system/files/2018-02/2017_09_18_ethical_consid_ct_with_minors_0.pdf

[23] Modi N, Vohra J, Preston J, et al. Guidance on clinical research involving infants, children and young people: An update for researchers and research ethics committees. Archives of Disease in Childhood. 2014;**99**:887-891

[24] European Commission, Directorate-General for Research and Innovation, Indicators for promoting and monitoring responsible research and innovation – Report from the Expert Group on policy indicators for responsible research and

innovation. Luxembourg: Publications Office; 2015. Available from: https://rri-tools.eu/ [Accessed: May 16, 2023]

[25] Council of Europe. Available from: https://www.coe.int/en/web/bioethics/guide-to-good-practice-concerning-the-participation-of-children [Accessed: May 16, 2023]

[26] United Nations. Universal Declaration of Human Rights. Geneva, Switzerland: UN General Assembly in Paris on 10 December 1948 during its 183rd plenary meeting. Article 25. 1948. Available from: https://www.un.org/en/about-us/universal-declaration-of-human-rights; 1948 [Accessed: May 16, 2023]

[27] European Union. Charter of Fundamental Rights. Article 24.Official Journal of the European Union C 303/17 - 14.12.2007. Luxembourg: Publications Office of the European Union; 2007. Available from: https://fra.europa.eu/en/eu-charter/title/title-iii-equality [Accessed: May 16, 2023]

[28] The National Commission for the Protection of Human Subjects of Biomedical and Behavioral Research. The Belmont Report. Ethical Principles and Guidelines for the Protection of Human Subjects of Research. The National Commission for the Protection of Human Subjects of Biomedical and Behavioral Research. Washington DC, USA: Government Printing Office; 1979. Available from: https://www.hhs.gov/ohrp/regulations-and-policy/belmont-report/read-the-belmont-report/index.html [Accessed: June 16, 2023]

[29] Partners in the BIOMED-II Project Basic Ethical Principles in Bioethics and Biolaw. Barcelona Declaration: Policy Proposals to the European Commission on Basic Ethical Principles in Bioethics and Biolaw. 1998. Available from: https://www.istitutobioetica.it/documenti-di-riferimento/documenti-di-riferimentoo/187-documenti/556-the-barcelona-declaration-on-policy-proposals-to-the-european-commission-on-basic-ethical-principles-in-bioethics-and-biolaw [Accessed: May 16, 2023]

[30] United Nations Educational, Scientific and Cultural Organization (UNESCO). Universal Declaration on Bioethics and Human Rights. Paris: UNESCO; 2005. Available from: https://www.unesco.org/en/legal-affairs/universal-declaration-bioethics-and-human-rights [Accessed: May 16, 2023]

[31] Council for International Organizations of Medical Sciences (CIOMS). Guideline 15. In: International Ethical Guidelines for Biomedical Research Involving Human Subjects. Geneva: CIOMS; 2016. pp. 57-59

[32] Luna F. Identifying and evaluating layers of vulnerability – A way forward. Developing World Bioethics. 2018;**19**(2):88

[33] Canadian Institutes of Health Research, Natural Sciences and Engineering Research Council of Canada, and Social Sciences and Humanities Research Council. Tri-Council, Policy Statement: Ethical Conduct for Research Involving Humans. Canada: Canadian Institutes of Health Research, Natural Sciences and Engineering Research Council of Canada, and Social Sciences and Humanities Research Council; 2022. Available from: https://ethics.gc.ca/eng/policy-politique_tcps2-eptc2_2022.html [Accessed: May 16, 2023]

[34] European Medicines Agency. International Council for Harmonisation (ICH) harmonised guideline integrated addendum to ICH E6(R1) (EMA/CHMP/ICH/135/1995): Guideline for Good Clinical Practice ICH E6(R2), Glossary.

2018. Available from: https://ichgcp.net/1-glossary [Accessed: May 16, 2023]

[35] Council for International Organizations of Medical Sciences (CIOMS). Guideline 16. In: International Ethical Guidelines for Biomedical Research Involving Human Subjects. Geneva: CIOMS; 2016. pp. 60-63

[36] McGregor KA, Ott MA. Banking the future: Adolescent capacity to consent to biobank research. Ethics and Human Research. 2019;**41**:15-22. DOI: 10.1002/eahr.500023

[37] Council for International Organizations of Medical Sciences (CIOMS). Guideline 9. In: International Ethical Guidelines for Biomedical Research Involving Human Subjects. Geneva: CIOMS; 2016. pp. 33-36

[38] Institute of Medicine. Understanding agreeing to children's participation in clinical research. In: Field MJ, Behrman RE, Institute of Medicine (US) Committee on Clinical Research Involving Children, editors. Ethical Conduct of Clinical Research Involving Children. Washington, DC: The National Academies; 2004

[39] Katz AL, Webb SA. AAP Committee on bioethics. Informed consent in decision-making in pediatric practice. Pediatrics. 2016;**138**:e20161485, [Technical Report]

[40] WHO. Working for a Brighter, healthier Future: How WHO Improves Health and Promotes Well-Being for the world's Adolescents. Geneva: World Health Organization; 2021. Licence: CC BY-NC-SA 3.0 IGO

[41] Hagan JF Jr, Shaw JS, Duncan P, editors. Bright Futures: Guidelines for the Health Supervision of Infants, Children, and Adolescents. 3rd ed. Elk Grove Village, IL: American Academy of Pediatrics; 2008

[42] Hein IM, De Vries MC, Troost PW, Meynen G, Van Goudoever JB, Lindauer RJ. Informed consent instead of assent is appropriate in children from the age of twelve: Policy implications of new findings on children's competence to consent to clinical research. BMC Medical Ethics. 2015;**16**:76. DOI: 10.1186/s12910-015-0067-z

[43] Hein IM, Troost PW, Lindeboom R, Benninga MA, Zwaan CM, Van Goudoever JB, et al. Accuracy of the MacArthur competence assessment tool for clinical research (MacCAT-CR) for measuring children's competence to consent to clinical research. JAMA Pediatrics. 2014;**168**:1147-1153

[44] European Network of Paediatric Research at the European Medicines Agency (EnprEMA). Informed Consent for Paediatric Clinical Trials in Europe 2015 Developed by the Working Group on Ethics. EnprEMA; 2019). Amsterdam, The Netherlands: European Medicines Agency; 2023. Available from: https://www.ema.europa.eu/en/documents/other/informed-consent-paediatricclinical-trials-europe-2015_en.pdf [Accessed: January 22, 2024]

[45] Lepola P, Kindred M, Giannuzzi V, et al. Informed consent and assent guide for paediatric clinical trials in Europe. Archives of Disease in Childhood. 2022;**107**:582-590

[46] National Health Service (NHS) Health Research Authority, UK. Research involving children. 2021. Available from: https://www.hra.nhs.uk/planning-and-improving-research/policies-standards-legislation/research-involving-children/ [Accessed: June 16, 2023]

[47] Hunter D, Pierscionek BK. Children, Gillick competency and consent for involvement in research. Journal of Medical Ethics. 2007;**33**:659-662

[48] Cotrim H, Granja C, Carvalho AS, Cotrim C, Martins R. Children's understanding of informed assents in research studies. Healthcare. 2021;**9**:871. DOI: 10.3390/healthcare9070871

[49] Joffe S, Cook E, Cleary P, Clark J, Weeks J. Quality of informed consent: A new measure of understanding among research subjects. Journal of the National Cancer Institute. 2001;**93**:139-147

[50] Soll D, Guraiib MM, Rollins NC, et al. Improving assent in health research: A rapid systematic review. BMC Medical Research Methodology. 2020;**20**:114. DOI: 10.1186/s12874-020-01000-3

[51] Tait AR, Geisser ME, Ray L, Hutchinson RJ, Voepel-Lewis T. Disclosing study information to children and adolescents: Is what they want, what their parents think they want? Academic Pediatrics. 2018;**18**(4):370-375. DOI: 10.1016/j.acap.2017.06.005

[52] Giesbertz NA, Bredenoord AL, van Delden JJ. Clarifying assent in pediatric research. European Journal of Human Genetics. 2014;**22**(2):266-269. DOI: 10.1038/ejhg.2013.119. Epub 2013 Jun 12

[53] Council for International Organizations of Medical Sciences (CIOMS). Appendix. In: International Ethical Guidelines for Biomedical Research Involving Human Subjects. Geneva: CIOMS; 2016. pp. 103-106

[54] Nuffield Council on Bioethics. Children and Clinical Research: Ethical Issues. London: Nuffield Council on Bioethics; 2015

[55] Council for International Organizations of Medical Sciences (CIOMS). Guideline 10. In: International Ethical Guidelines for Biomedical Research Involving Human Subjects. Geneva: CIOMS; 2016. pp. 37-39

[56] Comitato Nazionale per la Bioetica. Vaccini anti-covid-19 e adolescenti. Comitato Nazionale di Bioetica. Rome, Italy; 2021

[57] The National Commission for the Protection of Human Subjects of Biomedical Behavioral Research. Research Involving Children: Report Recommendations. DHEW Publication No. (OS) 77-0004. Washington, DC: U.S. Government Printing Office; 1977

[58] Fernandez CV, Bouffet E, Malkin D, Jabado N, O'Connell C, Avard D, et al. Attitudes of parents toward the return of targeted and incidental genomic research findings in children. Genetics in Medicine. 2014;**16**:633-640. DOI: 10.1038/gim.2013.201

[59] Matthijs G, Souche E, Alders M, Corveleyn A, Eck S, Feenstra I, et al. Guidelines for diagnostic next-generation sequencing. European Journal of Human Genetics. 2016;**24**(1):2-5. DOI: 10.1038/ejhg.2015.226. Epub 2015 Oct 28. Erratum in: Eur J Hum Genet. 2016 Oct;24(10):1515

[60] Knoppers BM, Avard D, Senecal K, Zawati MH. P3G international paediatrics platform members. Return of whole-genome sequencing results in paediatric research: A statement of the P3G international paediatrics platform. European Journal of Human Genetics. 2014;**22**:3-5. DOI: 10.1038/ejhg.2013.176

[61] Presidential Commission for the Study of Bioethical Issues. Anticipate and Communicate Ethical Management of Incidental and Secondary Findings

in the Clinical, Research, and Direct-to-Consumer Contexts. Washington,DC: Presidential Commission for the Study of Bioethical Issues; Dec 2013. Available from: https://papers.ssrn.com/sol3/papers.cfm?abstract_id=2459984 [Accessed: January 22, 2024]

[62] Comitato Nazionale per la Bioetica in. Managing "incidental findings" Genomic Investigations with New Technology Platforms. Rome, Italy: Comitato Nazionale per la Bioetica. Available from: https://bioetica.governo.it/media/4369/p123_2016_incidental-findings_en.pdf; 2016 [Accessed: June 22, 2023]

[63] Council of Europe. Additional Protocol to the Convention on Human Rights and Biomedicine, Concerning Biomedical Research. Strasbourg: Council of Europe; 2005. Article 27

[64] Federal Policy for the Protection of Human Subjects, 82 Fed. Reg. 7149 (Jan. 19, 2017)

[65] National Academies of Sciences, Engineering, and Medicine. Returning Individual Research Results to Participants: Guidance for a New Research Paradigm. Washington, DC: The National Academies Press; 2018. DOI: 10.17226/25094

[66] Council for International Organizations of Medical Sciences (CIOMS). Guidelines 11 and 12. In: International Ethical Guidelines for Biomedical Research Involving Human Subjects. Geneva: CIOMS; 2016. pp. 40-52. 2

[67] Global Alliance for Genomics and Health. Policy on Clinically Actionable Genomic Research Results 2021. Available from: https://www.ga4gh.org/wp-content/uploads/2021-Policy-on-Clinically-Actionable-Genomic-Research-Results.pdf

[68] Vears DF, Minion JT, Roberts SJ, Cummings J, Machirori M, Blell M, et al. Return of individual research results from genomic research: A systematic review of stakeholder perspectives. PLoS One. 2021;**16**:e0258646

[69] Bradbury AR, Patrick-Miller LJ, Egleston BL, DiGiovanni L, Brower J, Harris D, et al. Patient feedback and early outcome data with a novel tiered-binned model for multiplex breast cancer susceptibility testing. Genetics in Medicine. 2015;**18**:25-33. DOI: 10.1038/gim.2015.19. [PubMed: 25834950]

[70] Middleton A, Morley KI, Bragin E, Firth HV, Hurles ME, Wright CF, et al. Attitudes of nearly 7000 health professionals, genomic researchers and publics toward the return of incidental results from sequencing research. European Journal of Human Genetics: EJHG. 2016;**24**:21-29. DOI: 10.1038/ejhg.2015.58. [PubMed: 25920556]

[71] Ryan KA, De Vries RG, Uhlmann WR, Roberts JS, Gornick MC. Public's views toward return of secondary results in genomic sequencing: It's (almost) all about the choice. Journal of Genetic Counseling. 2017;**26**:1197-1212. DOI: 10.1007/s10897-017-0095-6

[72] Richer J, Laberge AM. Secondary findings from next-generation sequencing: What does actionable in childhood really mean? Genetics in Medicine. 2019;**21**:124-132. DOI: 10.1038/s41436-018-0034-4

[73] Hunter JE, Jenkins CL, Bulkley JE, Gilmore MJ, Lee K, Pak CM, etal. Clin Gen (2022). Clin Gen's pediatric actionability working group: Clinical actionability of secondary findings from genome-scale sequencing in children and adolescents. Genetics in Medicine, 24(6), 1328-1335. doi:10.1016/j.gim.2022.02.019

[74] Miller DT, Lee K, Chung WK, et al. ACMG SF v3.0 list for reporting of secondary findings in clinical exome and genome sequencing: A policy statement of the American College of Medical Genetics and Genomics (ACMG). Genetics in Medicine. 2021;**23**(8):1381-1390. Published correction appears in Genet Med. 2021;23(8):1582-1584. DOI: 10.1038/s41436-021-01172-3

[75] Green RC, Berg JS, Grody WW, et al. ACMG recommendations for reporting of incidental findings in clinical exome and genome sequencing. Genetics in Medicine. 2013;**15**:565-574

[76] Holm IA, Savage SK, Green RC, Juengst E, McGuire A, Kornetsky S, et al. Guidelines for return of research results from pediatric genomic studies: Deliberations of the Boston Children's Hospital Gene Partnership informed cohort oversight board. Genetics in Medicine. 2014;**16**(7):547-552. DOI: 10.1038/gim.2013.190

[77] Mackley MP, Fletcher B, Parker M, Watkins H, Ormondroyd E. Stakeholder views on secondary findings in whole-genome and whole-exome sequencing: A systematic review of quantitative and qualitative studies. Genetics in Medicine. 2017;**19**(3):283-293. DOI: 10.1038/gim.2016.109. Epub 2016 Sep 1

[78] Harris ED, Ziniel SI, Amatruda JG, et al. The beliefs, motivations, and expectations of parents who have enrolled their children in a genetic biorepository. Genetics in Medicine. 2012;**14**:330-337

[79] Sobel ME, Dreyfus JC, Dillehay McKillip K, Kolarcik C, Muller WA, Scott MJ, et al. Return of individual research results: A guide for biomedical researchers utilizing human biospecimens. The American Journal of Pathology. 2020;**190**(5):918-933. DOI: 10.1016/j.ajpath.2020.01.014

[80] Holm IA. Pediatric issues in return of results and incidental findings: Weighing autonomy and best interests. Genetic Testing and Molecular Biomarkers. 2017;**21**:155-158. DOI: 10.1089/gtmb.2016.0414

[81] Myers MF, Martin LJ, Prows CA. Adolescents' and parents' genomic testing decisions: Associations with age, race, and sex. Journal of Adolescent Health. 2020;**66**(3):288-295, ISSN 1054-139X. DOI: 10.1016/j.jadohealth.2019.08.028

[82] Wolf SM, Branum R, Koenig BA, Petersen GM, Berry SA, Beskow LM, et al. Returning a research participant's genomic results to relatives: Analysis and recommendations. The Journal of Law, Medicine & Ethics. 2015;**43**(3):440-463. DOI: 10.1111/jlme.12288

[83] EDPS, A Preliminary Opinion on data protection and scientific research at 19-20. 2020. Available from: https://edps.europa.eu/sites/edp/files/publication/20-01-06_opinion_research_en.pdf. [Accessed: June 16, 2023]

[84] Baldo et al. The alliance between genetic biobanks and patient organisations. Orphanet Journal of Rare Diseases. 2016;**11**:142. DOI: 10.1186/s13023-016-0526-7

[85] Kim EY. Biobanks as a treasury for precision medicine. Healthcare Informatics Research. 2021;**27**(2):93-94. DOI: 10.4258/hir.2021.27.2.93. Epub 2021 Apr 30

[86] Biobanking & Biomolecular Resources Research Infrastructure, Services & Support. Available from: https://www.bbmri-eric.eu/services-support/ [Accessed: June 16, 2023]

[87] Biobanking & Biomolecular Resources Research Infrastructure, Italian node. Towards good practice in biobanking for research. Available from: https://repository.bbmri.it/s/stC8Lc4kPDn2qQt

[88] Associazione Rete Italiana salute Dell'Età evolutivA (Rete IDEA), Ministero della Salute, Italia. Available from: https://retepediatricaidea.it/ [Accessed: June 16, 2023]

[89] Thorogood A, Dalpe G, Knoppers BM. Return of individual genomic research results: Are laws and policies keeping step? European Journal of Human Genetics: EJHG. 2019;**27**(4):535-546. DOI: 10.1038/s41431-018-0311-3

Section 3

Medical Perspectives

Chapter 9

Sexually Transmitted Disease Rates are Surging: A Matter of Life and Death

Shrikanth Sampath, Mahvish Renzu, Peter Clark, Joseph Kelly and Daniel Disandro

Abstract

After reaching historic lows decades ago, rates of sexually transmitted infections (STIs) have surged since 2020. Health officials claim that the pandemic was responsible for igniting this rise, citing a halt in testing, treatment, and surveillance of STIs as isolation began, and resources were reallocated to address coronavirus disease 2019 (COVID-19) issues. Others cite the overall shift in lawmaking since the early 2000s that has scaled back interventions geared toward controlling STI spread. Regardless of the root cause, this surge demands immediate attention due to the severe damage that these infections can cause, including infertility and pelvic inflammatory disease. In this paper, we examine this issue medically, socially, ethically, and from a public health perspective. The symptoms, treatments, complications, and testing strategies for syphilis, gonorrhea, and chlamydia are analyzed while highlighting at-risk groups and discussing mitigation strategies. The social implications of this current crisis are then explored, reviewing what approaches have been made for this issue so far. Next, we ground this issue in the harm reduction theory to advocate for the ethics of our proposed interventions. We conclude with recommendations at the individual, community, and federal levels to help reverse the surge in STIs and prevent further harm.

Keywords: STDs, social implications, ethics, economics, harm reduction

1. Introduction

The overall amount of sexually transmitted infections (STIs), namely syphilis, gonorrhea, and chlamydia continues to surge, specifically in the younger population. Combined cases of syphilis, gonorrhea, and chlamydia reached an all-time high after rising for the fifth year in a row. Between 2014 and 2018, cases of chlamydia, one of the most common STIs, increased by 15%. Although less prevalent overall, gonorrhea and syphilis increased by 35% and 50%, respectively [1]. Because these statistics only continue to rise, politically conservative policymakers remain set on limiting adolescent access to sexual health information and services because they believe that efforts to increase access to these resources will encourage sex among these populations; however, there is a range of research against this claim [1]. A shift in the methodology and approach to sexual health education in the youth is needed to turn back the trends in STIs.

Sexual relationships are a perfectly normal aspect of many young adult lives. In the United States, two-thirds of 18-year-olds have had sex; and by age 25, more than nine in 10 people will have had sex [1]. Thus, resources and programs aimed at preventing STIs through preventative education and access to treatment are a must-have aspect of approaching the surging STD rates in the United States.

After reaching a historic low in 2000 and 2001, primary and secondary syphilis rates have been steadily increasing every year, with an increase of 6.8% in 2019–2020 [1]. The US Midwest, Northeast, and the South saw an equal rise in both females and males. All racial groups witnessed a disproportionate increase in non-Hispanic American Indian/Alaska Native and non-Hispanic persons of multiple races.

Since 2000, men have seen an increase in primary and secondary (P&S) syphilis likely due to a rise in incidence among men who have sex with men (MSM), which appears to have slowed during 2019–2020. However, it is evident that MSM are affected disproportionately as they accounted for 53% of male P&S cases in 2020 with an increased syphilis rate witnessed in 18 states during the same period. Although women have a lower incidence of syphilis, it has substantially increased in recent years wherein the United States saw an increase of 147% in 2016–2020, suggesting a rapid increase in the heterosexual syphilis epidemic [1].

The congenital syphilis rate has been on the rise since 2008, with a massive 254% increase in the national rate from 2016 to 2020. This is reflective of the rise in syphilis in the reproductive women age group. There was a 24% increase in women aged 15–44 years [1].

Past years' data reveal some disparities in terms of age groups and racial minorities. The year 2020 saw 53% reported cases among adolescents and young adults and 32% of syphilis, gonorrhea, and chlamydia cases being non-Hispanic Black population despite making up only 12% of the US population. These expose the differences in access to sexual health care for the minority. Acknowledgment of health inequity is the first step toward empowering affected groups [2].

A mini epidemic of syphilis was seen from 1980 to 1990, with a peak in 1990, subsequently falling to lowest rates in 2000. According to the World Health Organization (WHO) estimate, in 2016, syphilis had a prevalence of 19.9 million and an incidence of 6.3 million [2].

The Centers for Disease Control and Prevention (CDC) report suggested recent increase in drug use could be a reason for increasing syphilis rates among women. Higher rates were seen among women who used methamphetamine, heroin, and intravenous (IV) drugs. Naturally, this increase heralded an increase in congenital syphilis with 2148 cases, 149 stillbirths, and infant deaths reported in 2020 [1, 2].

Another interesting trend is that 46% of MSM with syphilis were found to have coinfection with human immunodeficiency virus (HIV), in comparison to 8% in heterosexual men and 6% in women; men aged 25–29 years seemed to have the highest rates, and Black men seemed to be disproportionately affected with the incidence in 2020 as high as 57.7 per 100,000 versus 23.4 in Hispanic men and 11 in White men [3].

2. Methodology

This chapter is a multifaceted review of the current literature surrounding the rates of sexually transmitted diseases (STDs) and STIs to evaluate the current state of the crisis. We herein present the medical specifics of each disease covering historical perspectives, demographic data, transmission, symptoms, and treatment. In the analysis of the social aspect of this current crisis, we review and summarize various studies that provide a deeper context for our topic based on trends about national health care and political views. Our ethical analysis is similarly informed by national data, as we draw upon the work of renowned bioethicists to support our position in favor of our proposed initiatives as harm reduction techniques. Our public health recommendations are made in light of both evidence that similar interventions have worked in some capacity in the past and the guidelines from national and international health care institutions. The data were obtained from online databases and research articles.

3.Medical analysis

3.1 Syphilis

Syphilis is a sexually transmitted bacterial infection caused by *Treponema pallidum*. Humans have been plagued by the stigma of syphilis since the beginning of time when it was considered a disgraceful disease because of its means of infection. Historically, each country blamed its neighbors for the outbreak. Germany, Italy, and the United Kingdom called it the "French disease", Russians called it the "Polish disease", the Polish named it the "German disease", and so on [4].

Syphilis is also marred by the infamous Tuskegee study (1932 to 1972) that disregarded bioethics by withholding treatment for syphilis to 431 Black men enrolled after it became available during the study period and providing insufficient information regarding the study to obtain informed consent [5].

3.1.1 Symptoms

Syphilis is also known as "The Great Pretender" because the symptoms mimic several other diseases. Progression of syphilis can last from a few weeks to months to years, advancing through primary, secondary, and tertiary stages. The primary stage is characterized by chancres, which are round, firm, and painless open sores, typically found in unnoticeable places such as the vagina or anus. The source can last from 3 to 6 weeks and will heal regardless of treatment. If left untreated, syphilis will progress to the secondary stage [4, 6]. The secondary stage is marked by a non-itchy rash on skin or mucous membranes, which originate from one area of the body and spread to another. On many occasions, this rash may be very faint to notice. One may also develop a condyloma lata lesion, which is a raised lesion that develops around moist and warm areas such as the axilla, genitals, or mouth. Patients may also experience sore throat, fever, enlarged lymph nodes, hair loss, headaches, or fatigue. Similar to primary syphilis, secondary syphilis symptoms will resolve without treatment, but the disease itself will progress to latent syphilis likely followed by tertiary syphilis [4, 6]. Latent syphilis is the period without any visible signs/symptoms and can last for years [4, 6]. However, tertiary syphilis is one of the most potentially fatal stages, which can develop 10 to 30 years after the infection, affecting multiple organs, such as the brain, nerves, heart, liver, eyes, and bones [4, 6].

Other dangers associated with syphilis include its effects on pregnant mothers and their children. It can be transmitted from a pregnant woman to her unborn baby. Testing is usually recommended during the first prenatal visit and sometimes at the third trimester and delivery as well. People living in areas with higher syphilis rates may also need testing [4, 6]. Multiple sex partners, late prenatal care, methamphetamine use, incarceration, and homelessness all predispose individuals to syphilis during pregnancy. The longer a pregnant woman has syphilis, the higher the chances are for stillbirths. Pregnant women with untreated syphilis experience an infant death rate of up to 40% [4, 6]. Untreated babies who contract syphilis from their mothers can develop seizures, experience developmental delays, or even die. Hence, it is paramount to treat infected mothers with penicillin, as it prevents transmission in 98% of cases [4, 6].

3.1.2 Testing

Testing comprises two strategies: screening and diagnosis. Screening is performed on those who are asymptomatic but at a high risk of infection, whereas diagnostic tests are performed on those who have signs or symptoms of the disease or test positive during the screening. It is important to understand the type of patients we need to test. Knowing that syphilis presents widely, one should have a low threshold for testing. Patients presenting with classic signs such as genital ulcers, rash involving trunk and extremities, and general weakness must be tested. Additionally, a sexually active person with a rash in the palms and soles and an undiagnosed genital ulcer should be tested.

Tests available for syphilis are serologic tests and direct tests. These two tests alone or in combination are used to screen and diagnose individuals [6]. Serologic tests help in obtaining a presumptive diagnosis of syphilis and are usually used in conjunction with nontreponemal tests, which measure the serum reactivity of infected patients to a cardiolipin-cholesterol-lecithin antigen. Despite being nonspecific and nondefinitive, they are inexpensive, easy to perform, and useful following response to therapy. Thus, it has been traditionally used as an initial screening tool for syphilis. Examples of non-treponemal tests are the rapid plasma reagin (RPR) test, the Venereal Disease Research Laboratory (VDRL) test, and the toluidine red unheated serum test (TRUST). These tests are semiquantitative and wane over a period even without treatment. They are reported as titers, and the changing titer denotes a response to therapy [6].

Treponemal tests, on the other hand, are complex and expensive tests. Once nontreponemal tests are positive, treponemal tests are performed and hence are traditional confirmatory tests. However, the advent of advanced technologies has facilitated ease of use, simplicity, and automation, increasing their use as an initial screening test, which is now referred to as reverse screening. Examples of these tests include the fluorescent treponemal antibody absorption (FTA-ABS) test, the *T. pallidum* particle agglutination assay (TPPA) test, the *T. pallidum* enzyme immunoassay (TP-EIA) test, chemiluminescence immunoassay (CIA), and microhemagglutination test for antibodies to keep *T. pallidum* (MHA-TP). These tests detect the antibodies developed by the patient against specific treponemal antigens and hence are more specific than nontreponemal tests. They are reported either as "reactive" or "nonreactive" and usually remain positive for the rest of their lives [6].

The tests that definitively confirm the presence of *T. pallidum* are called direct tests. These include darkfield microscopy/direct fluorescent antibody testing and polymerase chain reaction (PCR) tests. The former needs advanced equipment and expertise to perform and hence are not routinely used by clinicians. However, some labs have developed PCR tests to detect the bacteria in clinical specimens. One limitation of these, though, is that they have low sensitivity and might detect dead organisms too [6].

Considering all the factors described above, serologic tests are frequently used to make a presumptive diagnosis. Traditionally, nontreponemal tests (e.g., RPR) followed by a treponemal test (e.g., FTA-ABS) have been used for diagnosis. However, in recent years when treponemal tests have become easy to perform as mentioned above, a reverse algorithm is becoming popular. The CDC was the first one to describe this in 2008. An example would be performing TP-EIA followed by RPR or VDRL [6].

3.1.3 Treatment

The data on the treatment of early syphilis support the use of a single intramuscular injection of 2.4 million U of benzathine penicillin G, with studies reporting 90–100% treatment success rates. The value of multiple-dose treatment of early syphilis is uncertain, especially in HIV-infected individuals. Less evidence is available regarding therapy for late and late latent syphilis. Following treatment, nontreponemal serologic titers should decline in a stable pattern, but a significant proportion of patients may remain seropositive (the "serofast state").6 Serologic response to treatment should be evident by 6 months in early syphilis but is generally slower (12–24 months) for latent syphilis. Evidence defining treatment for HIV-infected persons and for pregnant women is limited, but available data support penicillin as the first-line therapy [5].

While penicillin remains the drug of choice to treat syphilis, doxycycline to treat early and late latent syphilis is an acceptable alternate option if penicillin cannot be used. There are very limited data regarding the impact of additional antibiotic doses on serologic responses in serofast patients and no data on the impact of additional antibiotic courses on long-term clinical outcomes [7]. Here, we will summarize the treatment protocols as listed by the CDC.

3.1.3.1 Adults

3.1.3.1.1 Primary and secondary syphilis

A single dose of 2.4 million units of intramuscular benzathine penicillin G has been effective in healing the rashes and preventing sexual transmission and late sequelae. Additional antibiotics have not been known to enhance the above-mentioned treatment regimen [5].

3.1.3.1.2 Tertiary syphilis

If a patient does not have cardiovascular syphilis, gummas, has absent CSF or clinical findings of neurosyphilis, and is not allergic to penicillin, then the protocol dictates 2.4 million units of intramuscular benzathine penicillin G given once weekly for a total of three doses [5].

3.1.3.1.3 Latent syphilis

Treatment of this stage is meant to prevent complications rather than treat, as latent syphilis is not sexually transmissible. Penicillin is known to be the treatment of choice here as well; however, the choice of duration of treatment has limited evidence. Early latent syphilis is treated with one dose of 2.4 million units of intramuscular benzathine penicillin, whereas latent syphilis needs once weekly dose of 2.4 million units of intramuscular benzathine penicillin for a total of three doses [5].

3.1.3.2 Penicillin allergy

Although penicillin remains the mainstay and most effective medication for the treatment of syphilis, penicillin allergy necessitates the use of effective alternatives. In the case of primary and secondary syphilis, oral doxycycline 100 mg BID for 14 days or oral tetracycline 500 mg 4 times a day for 14 days can be used. For latent syphilis, 28 days of the above-stated regimen is effective. Tertiary syphilis patients allergic to penicillin need a referral to infectious disease [8].

3.1.3.3 Pregnant women

The treatment regimen for pregnant women is the same for adults for their respective stages but with certain special considerations. Those with penicillin allergy should undergo desensitization and be treated with their recommended doses of penicillin. Allergy testing through skin tests and graded oral dose challenges can help identify those at risk [9].

3.1.3.4 Syphilis with HIV infection

Treatment for this population group is the same for adults without HIV for their respective stages. Those with HIV and latent syphilis must be monitored closely for treatment response at 6, 12, 18, and 24 months [10].

3.2 Gonorrhea

Gonorrhea is a sexually transmitted infection caused by *Neisseria gonorrhea* and is the second most common bacterial STI after chlamydia. In fact, these infections often occur together. It spreads through semen or vaginal secretions during sexual intercourse, oral or anal sex, and the sharing of sex toys with someone who is infected. Additionally, because symptoms often go unnoticed, it is easily transmissible to partners [11].

3.2.1 Symptoms

Females are often affected and more than 70% are asymptomatic. Some patients can have cervicitis, urethritis, pelvic inflammatory disease (PID) and even complications of pregnancy. In cervicitis, when symptoms do occur, they emerge in the form of vaginal itching and/or pus discharge. On cervical examination, one may see frank pus and friable mucosa [12]. In urethritis, the female might be asymptomatic or can have burning urination, urinary urgency, or urinary frequency. PID is a serious complication of cervicitis where a patient can have abdominal tenderness, a tender uterus, and cervical motion tenderness, among other symptoms. PID can be further complicated in the form of perihepatitis, also called Fitz Hugh Curtis syndrome [12]. One of the major areas of impact is pregnancy where the mother with gonorrhea can have complications such as preterm birth, small for gestational age infants, and low birth weight [12].

Males often contract urethritis or epididymitis. They present with penile discharge and dysuria, unilateral testicular swelling, and pain in the epididymitis [12].

3.2.2 Testing

Women less than 24 years old who are sexually active and women over 25 years old who are at increased risk of infection are recommended by the United States Preventive Services Task Force (USPSTF) to be screened for gonorrhea. Insufficient evidence regarding benefit versus harm exists for testing men [13].

Historically, the gold standard test for gonorrhea was culture. It is a low-cost method and has a sensitivity of 72–95%, which increases to 95–100% in the hands of experienced lab technicians. DNA extracted from the cultures has become the best method to perform genomic analysis because clinical specimens tend to contain either not enough DNA or have DNA from other bacteria and human cells [13].

Microscopy is the method of choice in resource-deficient settings where gram-stained samples are visualized under a microscope. Sensitivity and specificity can differ based on the site of sample collection but usually range between 89 and 98% for urethral swabs. It is not suitable for specimens obtained from the pharynx or rectum [13].

The nucleic acid amplification test (NAAT) is the diagnostic method of choice in resource-rich environments. It allows noninvasive testing because the specimen needed is either urine or self-collected vaginal swabs. Storage and transportation of specimens are easy because viable organisms are not required for NAAT [14]. Other advantages include rapid results, automation, and the ability to detect other STI pathogens such as chlamydia. However, the disadvantage is that one cannot obtain antimicrobial resistance data and strain characterization through this method, which removes the ability to assess resistance patterns and strain prevalence [14].

3.2.3 Treatment

Uncomplicated gonococcal infection affecting the pharynx, urethra, rectum, or cervix is treated with a single intramuscular shot of ceftriaxone at 500 mg if the patient weighs less than 150 kg and 1 g of ceftriaxone if the patient weighs more than 150 kg according to CDC. In case of allergy, a single intramuscular dose of gentamicin (240 mg) and a single dose of oral azithromycin (2 g) are effective [15]. If intramuscular ceftriaxone cannot be given or is not available, a single dose of oral cefixime (800 milligrams) can be given. Recent sexual partners who are engaged in sexual activity less than 60 days before the onset of symptoms in the patient are to be referred for evaluation and testing [15].

3.3 Chlamydia

Chlamydia is currently the most common bacterial STI. It is caused by *Chlamydia trachomatis* and reportedly affects around 1.5 million people a year. Chlamydia usually does not have signs and symptoms; hence, it goes unreported in most cases. People who are more likely to contract this infection are teens or young adults between 15 and 24 years old, men who have sex with men, and members of the Black and Hispanic populations [16]. It is transmitted through oral, vaginal, or rectal intercourse with an infected person. Additionally, a pregnant mother can pass it on to the infant during childbirth [17].

3.3.1 Symptoms

About 70% of women and 50% of men remain asymptomatic [18]. Common symptoms include cervicitis, pelvic inflammatory disease, urethritis, hepatitis, epididymitis, proctitis, prostatitis, reactive arthritis, conjunctivitis, ammonia, pharyngitis, and lymphogranuloma venereum [19].

3.3.2 Testing

CDC recommends screening any symptomatic patient. Other than that, certain high-risk groups are screened as they demonstrate high prevalence. These groups are sexually active women younger than 25 years old, pregnant women, and men and women with multiple sexual partners.

When the cell culture method is used, samples are typically collected from the anus, urethra, cervix, or conjunctiva. However, cell culture is rarely used today, as it is laborious, time-consuming, has average sensitivity, and has specific storage and transportation requirements. Nevertheless, they are useful in determining antimicrobial sensitivity and in cases of sexual assault where you need the highest level of specificity [20].

Nucleic acid amplification tests (NAAT) have become the gold standard of testing because of the ease of storage and transportation, non-dependency on viable pathogens, and specificity comparable to culture [20].

One drawback to NAATs is that they were centrally performed in a laboratory, which meant that samples would be sent to the laboratory, and once the results were generated, they were sent back to the physician. This meant that the patient had to make two visits to know the results. This is where rapid diagnostic tests (RDTs) became popular, as they were point-of-care tests providing results within minutes, enabling initiation of antibiotics immediately after. They work on the principle of immunochromatography [20]. Overall, though, NAATs are most sensitive and specific and are the test of choice.

3.3.3 Treatment

Chlamydia can cause serious complications such as PID and infertility. In men, chlamydia and gonorrhea often coexist and require diagnosis and treatment. Partners of affected patients should be tested, instructed to avoid sex for 1 week after starting the therapy, instructed to consider an HIV test, and provided counseling regarding high-risk behaviors [19].

Oral doxycycline (100 mg) twice per day for 7 days is the recommended regimen in adolescents and adults. Alternatively, one can use a single dose of oral azithromycin (1 gram) or oral levofloxacin (500 mg) daily for 7 days [19].

Abstinence from sex is advised while being on the 7-day therapy or until symptoms resolve, and all the sexual partners should be treated as well. Sexual partners must undergo screening and treatment if they had sex within 60 days of symptom emergence in the affected individual [21].

3.4 MSM and syphilis

Men who have sex with men (MSM) and syphilis have a very interesting relationship. They are one of the most disproportionately affected groups in several countries, and many factors are contributory to this incidence and prevalence.

In the subsequent decades after the introduction of penicillin for the treatment of syphilis in the 1940s, rates went up in the MSM group. The 1980s witnessed HIV/AIDs that was coupled with a rise in syphilis rates, hence exposing the potentiation effect of both STIs. The 1990s saw a sharp fall in syphilis rates as the CDC pushed for elimination. However, this was short-lived, as the rates resurged in the 2000s, and this time, they were associated with methamphetamine use. Between 2020 and 2021, 36% of syphilis cases reported were from MSM and bisexual men [22]. A meta-analysis of the data from 2000 to 2020 revealed a 7.5% global pooled prevalence of syphilis among MSM [23].

Behavioral aspects that drove these changes were unsafe sex, anonymous sex, higher usage of dating apps, visiting bathhouses, and as stated above, the use of crystal methamphetamine. In addition to this, because of the stigma and discrimination associated with homosexuality, MSM may either not disclose their sexual identity or avoid seeking testing and treatment.

Syphilis in MSM remains a major infectious disease conundrum. To address the disparity and to tackle high syphilis rates in MSM, health care needs to implement enhanced screening for those at increased risk every 3–6 months, improve access to testing, address discrimination, tailor counseling, advocate condom use, and educate regarding pre-exposure prophylaxis.

By addressing syphilis in this population, we can work toward reducing the overall burden of this preventable infection [24]. The CDC now has a new recommendation that can dramatically reduce the rates of certain STIs in MSM, bisexual men, and transgender women. A study demonstrated that a single dose of oral doxycycline (200 mg) when taken within 24–72 hr. of unprotected anal sex is an effective post-exposure prophylaxis. The study found to reduce the incidence of chlamydia and syphilis by 70 and 73%, respectively [25].

3.5 STIs and minorities

Health equity stands for equal chance at health regardless of race, sex, ethnicity, income, gender, religion, sexual identity, and disability. Among the above, race and ethnicity play a major role in accessing health care. It is noted that certain racial or ethnic minorities have a higher prevalence of STI. What is important to understand that this is not due to their heritage or ethnicity but the factors that affect them specifically, such as poverty, lower employment rates, and lower education rates, which make it harder for marginalized groups to stay healthy.

Low socioeconomic status restricts access to quality health care. Many minorities have lower trust in the health care system because of the fear of discrimination from doctors and other health care workers. With all of this, once STD rates rise within a community, sexually active groups are now more likely to meet infected individuals from their community [26].

It is crucial to establish specialized prevention and screening measures catered to the requirements of particular communities to overcome these racial discrepancies. This could entail expanding access to testing and treatment, offering care that is culturally sensitive, addressing social and economic risk factors, and including partnering with communities in prevention initiatives. Addressing racial disparities in STIs is crucial for achieving health equity and enhancing the general health of all communities.

3.6 Implications

Every day, over 1 million people acquire STIs [27]. According to the Centers for Disease Control and Prevention (CDC), gonorrhea, syphilis, and chlamydia combined accounted for more than 2.4 million cases in 2018, and 1.8 million cases in 2013, with half of these cases noted in the youth [28].

The recent increase in STIs is a concerning public health issue that has to be addressed immediately. The increase in STDs has significant ramifications for persons of all ages, public health organizations, and the society. A few of these are listed below:

3.6.1 Health risks

The following significant, sometimes fatal side effects can result from STDs: malignancy, infertility, ectopic pregnancy, spontaneous abortion, stillbirth, low birth weight, chronic pain, neurologic impairment, and even death. The rise in STD rates means that more people are at risk of experiencing these health problems.

3.6.1.1 Women

There exists an array of reasons for women being more prone than men to experience STD problems. Female biology predisposes women to a higher chance of contracting STI when exposed to one. It is easier for many STIs to travel from male to female than vice versa. Women are also more likely to experience delayed identification and treatment of STIs, which raises the likelihood of negative outcomes [29].

Salpingitis and infertility are two widely known sequelae of STIs. *Trichomonas vaginalis*, *Mycoplasma genitalium*, and other bacteria could possibly cause tubal damage and other potential infertility causes. Furthermore, a number of STI infections are linked to a higher risk of miscarriage and infant mortality [30].

The most prevalent reportable disease in the United States is *C. trachomatis*, with an estimated 3 million infections per year among the population [31]. An asymptomatic chlamydia infection can induce a fallopian tube infection. Infertility may result from irreversible damage to the fallopian tubes, uterus, and surrounding tissues brought on by PID and "silent" infection in the upper vaginal tract [32]. Gonococcal PID has been demonstrated to be a significant contributor to fallopian tube damage, significantly raising a woman's chance of tubal factor infertility (TFI) similar to chlamydial PID. Clinical manifestations of acute PID are present in 10–19% of women with cervical *N. gonorrhoeae* infections [32].

Syphilis, with an incidence of over 10 million cases per year, dramatically affects pregnancy; almost one-third of untreated pregnant women lose their child to stillbirth or neonatal mortality. The remaining one-third are born with congenital syphilis, which leads to another 300,000 perinatal deaths every year [32].

3.6.1.2 Men

Men can be rendered infertile by chlamydia and other STIs that can cause complications such as orchitis, particularly epididymo-orchitis, and prostatitis [33]. Studies on animals have demonstrated that chlamydial infection results in a large loss of germ cells due to spermatogonial apoptosis, leaving only Sertoli cells in the most damaged seminiferous tubules, which also exhibit elevated apoptotic activity [34]. Neisseria can cause vestibulitis, penile edema, prostatitis, orchitis, or chronic epididymitis if the disease is untreated [35].

Acute epididymo-orchitis frequently causes poor semen quality and reduced sperm motility and count. In addition, if ascending infections are not appropriately treated, they may result in testicular injury or azoospermia because of blockage.

However, despite advancements, pelvic inflammatory disease is still a problem due to the infeasibility of programs designed to prevent pelvic inflammatory disease in a large portion of the developing world and the suboptimal reproductive outcomes among treated patients [36].

Preventing and controlling STIs caused by *C. trachomatis* or *N. gonorrhoeae* is the most crucial public health approach for the prevention of pelvic inflammatory disease. Based on evidence from randomized controlled trials showing that detecting and treating cervical *C. trachomatis* infection can reduce a woman's risk of pelvic inflammatory disease by roughly 30–50% over a year, numerous high-income countries have put in place programs to screen and treat women for asymptomatic *C. trachomatis* infection [37].

3.6.2 Economic costs

In the United States, STDs have a considerable impact on morbidity and death. They range from conditions that, for the most part, only result in brief discomfort and inconvenience to conditions that shorten life expectancy, affect fertility, or cause long-term morbidity [29]. The rising STD prevalence could impose a strain on public health budgets and health care systems because of the high cost of treating STDs. This may result in higher health care expenses and less access to care for other medical conditions. Eight major STIs' direct medical expenses are thought to cost the US $16.7 billion. This estimate considers the costs of gonorrhea, chlamydia, syphilis, trichomoniasis, hepatitis B, illnesses brought on by sexually transmitted HPV, genital HSV-2 infections, and HIV infection in the United States in 2008 [38].

3.6.3 Social stigma

"The shroud of stigma, shame, and anxiety," which affects both patients and health care professionals, is another underlying factor in the epidemic and one that continues to thwart efforts to control STDs [39]. Because STDs are frequently stigmatized and linked to unfavorable stereotypes, those who get them may experience prejudice and shame. As a result, patients may be reluctant to admit they have issues, ignore them, or attribute them to other factors. Additionally, this stigma may discourage individuals from getting tested and treated, which may further the spread of STDs.

3.6.4 Sex education

Comprehensive sex education has been demonstrated to alter many of the behaviors, attitudes, and beliefs that have been linked to an increased risk of contracting STIs [40]. The increase in STD incidence emphasizes the need for more thorough sexual education programs in communities and schools. These initiatives can promote testing and treatment, disseminate knowledge about safe sexual practices, and assist to stop the spread of STDs. Families, communities, and several other facets of society must work together to support teenagers in making healthy decisions, and schools play a crucial role in this process [41].

3.6.5 Public health policies

To counteract the rising STD prevalence, governments may need to adopt or amend public health policies and programs. This might entail boosting financing for screening and treatment, expanding access to medical care, and putting more potent preventative measures in place. Given that structural interventions, including policies, have the potential to reach a large number of people with less effort and expense than many other interventions, they may be of particular importance to public health. In general, the rising incidence of STDs has a big impact on people, communities, and society. A complex strategy involving education, prevention, and therapy is necessary to address the problem.

3.7 STDs and HIV

HIV infection risk may be higher for those with STDs. One explanation is that actions such as not using condoms, having several partners, or dating anonymous people frequently put someone at risk for various illnesses. In addition, since STDs and

HIV frequently co-occur, having an STD means that the person who contracted it may also have HIV or other STDs at risk. Finally, an STD or inflammation may cause HIV infection that would have been prevented by healthy skin [42]. It is commonly recognized that STDs can greatly raise a person's risk of contracting HIV, but many individuals are still unaware of why this is the case or how STDs can easily enable infection, even in otherwise low-risk situations such as oral sex. The likelihood of contracting one of these illnesses is increased by the fact that many of them go misdiagnosed.

Defensive cells such as CD4 and CD8 T-cells are enlisted to the front lines in a localized infection, such as STD. The "killer" CD8 T-cells are guided by the "helper" CD4 T-cells to neutralize the infection. Ironically, HIV preferentially targets CD4 cells for infection, the very cells designed to signal an attack. Consequently, the likelihood that HIV will be able to get beyond the body's first line of defenses increases with the strength of the pathogenic onslaught and the recruitment of target cells [43]. In general, people who have other STIs including chlamydia, gonorrhea, and syphilis are more likely to get HIV if they have unprotected sexual contact with a partner who is infected. Co-infection with HIV and syphilis is prevalent and affects patient groups with similar characteristics. All patients with syphilis should be provided with HIV testing, and all HIV-positive patients should get routine syphilis screenings [44]. This co-infection has a detrimental effect on immunological recovery and antiretroviral efficacy [45].

A meta-analysis and systematic review performed by Meng Yin Wu et al. showed that there was a twofold increase in the incidence of HIV in patients already infected with syphilis. This could stem from high-risk behaviors that are common for the acquisition of STIs such as unsafe sex and IV drug abuse. As mentioned earlier, certain ethnic and racial groups might not seek or get quality health care because of stigma or discrimination that then extends into HIV going undiagnosed for a longer time or the continuation of high-risk behaviors [46].

Other studies found a 19.6% prevalence of other STIs in those who tested positive for HIV. Erbelding et al. found that HIV transmission is soon followed by another STD where he demonstrated that men took 415 days and women took 176 days to contract a new STI following the diagnosis of HIV [47]. HIV and syphilis co-infection has seen a rise in recent years after a decline during the COVID-19 pandemic. Most recent numbers indicate a tripling of prevalence in the United States from 2013 to 2018, a 50% increase in Europe from 2009 to 2018, a doubling in Canada from 2008 to 2017, and a 135% increase in Australia from 2013 to 2017 [47].

There are several contributory reasons for this increase. Earlier in the 1990s, because of the scare of HIV infection, individuals reduced high-risk sex behaviors, which in turn led to a fall in syphilis rates. However, once antiretroviral therapy came into existence and improved life expectancy and quality of life, there was a resurgence of syphilis in the past 2 decades mainly in the United States, Europe, Canada, Australia, and China. This has been further compounded by the availability of pre-exposure prophylaxis, the increasing trend of casual sex through dating apps, drug use during sex, and even a reduction in public health spending in several regions. Syphilis rates are rising across a wide range of groups in several geographic locations. Modern clinicians must be especially vigilant of syphilis in high-risk patients, such as those who are MSM or have risk factors for HIV acquisition [48].

3.7.1 Complications

Several patients with STDs often do not present any symptoms [49]. However, if untreated, there may be negative long-term side effects that could be disastrous, such as:

- Syphilis, in its advanced and complicated stages, causes neurosyphilis that leads to dementia, tabes dorsalis and sensory deficits; ocular syphilis that can present as anterior or posterior uveitis; cardiac syphilis that causes aortic aneurysm and coronary arteritis; and when passed onto the neonate during birth, it causes congenital syphilis.

- Blindness: *C. trachomatis* infection causes trachoma, an eye condition that can result in blindness. About 1.9 million people worldwide have blindness or visual impairment as a result of this public health issue. Blindness brought on by trachoma is permanent [50]. Other syphilis and gonorrhea, two STDs in particular, can induce eye infections that, if ignored, can impair eyesight or even result in blindness.

- Hepatitis B and C are sexually transmitted diseases that can result in chronic hepatitis, which can harm the liver and even result in cancer.

- Cancers: Hepatitis B and C can raise the chance of liver cancer, and HPV (human papillomavirus) can cause cervical cancer. Most malignancies of the cervix, vagina, vulva, anus, and penis are now thought to be caused by certain forms of sexually transmitted human papillomavirus.

- PID, or pelvic inflammatory disease, which can affect a woman's fallopian tubes and cause sterility.

- Tubal pregnancy (growth of the fetus in the fallopian tube)

- Congenital birth defects

- Death

4. Social implications

In the early months of the COVID-19 pandemic, there was a decrease in the number of reported cases of STDs such as syphilis, gonorrhea, and chlamydia, yet the prevalence of these diseases surged toward the latter half of 2020. Rather than a true decrease in the number of infections, it seems more likely that this decrease was instead due to a lack of adequate reporting measures amid the initial public health COVID-19 response. This breakdown of reporting methods of the public health infrastructure for STD reporting was influenced by several factors as follows: reduced frequency of in-person health care services as routine visits decreased ...; diversion of public health staff from STD work to respond to the COVID-19 pandemic; STD test and laboratory supply shortages; lapses in health insurance coverage due to unemployment; and telemedicine practices that led to some infections not being captured in the national data [51]. Not all groups were affected equally, rather, the majority of this increase was within racial and ethnic minority groups, homosexual and bisexual men, and the nation's youth.

These trends are not unusual in health care, rather, these populations experience disparities in health care generally due to longstanding social and economic factors such as poverty and health insurance status... [which] create barriers, increase health risks, and often result in worse health outcomes for some people [51]. Similar to attempting to promote social justice and equity in other health care disparities, public health officials and policymakers must understand how structural and institutional barriers lead to some individuals receiving a disproportionately low amount of care and therefore poor health outcomes. Over the last 50 years, there has been a common regression in the number of health care facilities available to poverty-stricken areas because hospitals and doctors are following privately insured patients to more affluent areas rather than remaining grounded in communities having the greatest health care needs [52]. This drop has been significant. The number of hospitals in 52 major cities in the United States has fallen from its peak of 781 in 1970 to 426 in 2010, a drop of 46% [52]. This lack of access to primary care for these vulnerable populations leads to a disproportionately low number of intervention and therefore higher rates of STDs and STIs. A study to determine the relationship between basic health care access and the rates of sexually transmitted relations found that by increasing the percentage of residents with a primary care provider was associated with a 39% lower STI risk [53]. Overall, greater health care access generally is correlative with fewer STDs and STIs. Further research should look to evaluate the pathways through which health care access influences STIs and take action to combat these pathways on a structural level.

As the combined cases of syphilis, gonorrhea, and chlamydia among young adults in the United States reach new record highs each year, conservative policymakers maintain their intent to limit the number of sexual education that our youth receives [1]. There is a broad range of factors to be blamed for the increasing prevalence of STIs among the youth including the following: decreased condom use; declining local, state, and federal investment in STI programs; expanding sexual networks facilitated by dating apps; the rise of antibiotic-resistant strains of certain STIs; and, potentially, increased testing [1]. One intervention that could help to mitigate the effects of nearly all other factors is the increase in sexual education, equipping individuals with the skills necessary to foster healthy relationships and healthily express their sexual nature, understanding consent, and good sexual habits [1]. The current all-or-nothing mindset that conservative policymakers have toward sexual education, which is the abstinence-only option, does not align with the reality of adolescents' sexual activity and does not prepare them for sex in adulthood [1]. To fully prepare this generation to be capable of managing their sexual relationships in a safely and healthily, a complete sexual education program that stresses the importance of practicing safe sex is a requirement for the long-term fight against STIs among adolescents.

5. Ethical analysis

5.1 Harm reduction as practical ethical justification

The STD epidemic in the United States shows no signs of slowing. Reported cases of sexually transmitted infections (STIs) chlamydia, gonorrhea, and syphilis all increased between 2020 and 202, reaching a total of more than 2.5 million reported cases according to the CDC's final surveillance data. To reverse this trend, CDC is calling for more groups from the local health care industry and public health sectors to contribute to STI prevention and innovation efforts [54]. Various recommendations have been proposed to control the spread of STDs: increasing condom availability and use; developing new safe and effective vaccines, adult voluntary medical male circumcision, microbicides, partner treatment, information, education and counseling especially among the minority populations; increasing resources for screening and treatment; increasing funding and access to quality sexual health care services; and doing advanced scientific research exploring new interventions. Many of these recommendations are being proposed as an ethical way to decrease the STD epidemic as part of the harm reduction technique. Harm reduction is an approach focused on minimizing the negative results that go hand-in-hand with drug abuse and risky sexual behavior [55, 56]. Harm reduction techniques have both medical and ethical impact on the individual and society. Harm reduction techniques accept the individuals as they are while also tailoring that person's treatment to fit his or her needs [57]. Furthermore, there are certain principles that are quintessential to an understanding of harm reduction, as listed by the Harm Reduction Coalition as follows:

- Accepts, for better or worse, that licit and illicit drug use and risky sexual behavior are part of our world and chooses to work to minimize its harmful effects rather than simply ignore or condemn them.

- Understands drug use and risky sexual behavior as a complex, multifaceted phenomenon that encompasses a continuum of behaviors from severe abuse to total abstinence and acknowledges that some ways of using drugs and engaging in sexual relations are clearly safer than others.

- Establishes quality of individual and community life and well-being—not necessarily cessation of all drug use and sexual behavior—as the criteria for successful interventions and policies.

- Calls for the nonjudgmental, noncoercive provision of services and resources to people who use drugs and engage in risky sexual behavior and the communities in which they live in order to assist them in reducing attendant harm.

- Ensures that drug users and those with a history of drug use and those individuals who are HIV or have STDs routinely have a real voice in the creation of programs and policies designed to serve them.

- Affirms drugs users and those who engage in risky sexual behavior themselves as the primary agents of reducing the harms of their drug use and sexual behavior and seeks to empower these individuals to share information and support each other in strategies that meet their actual conditions of use and behavior.

- Recognizes that the realities of poverty, class, racism, social isolation, past trauma, sex-based discrimination, and other social inequalities affect both people's vulnerability to and capacity for effectively dealing with drug-related harm and risky sexual behavior.

- Does not attempt to minimize or ignore the real and tragic harm and danger associated with licit and illicit drug use and risky sexual behavior [55].

The recommendations proposed in this paper to end the current STD epidemic have the potential to be used as a harm reduction agent in and of itself as it can save lives. Furthermore, many individuals who become STD infected did not receive necessary medical education to increase STD prevention and have become infected. Advocating for our proposed recommendations that include increasing resources, decreasing stigmatization, increasing better quality of health care services, and decreasing out-of-pocket expenses possibly could save many preventable infections and even deaths. If we value human life as sacred, we must find a way to prevent these deaths. Creating a national strategic plan, which increases health care resources especially among the minority populations, encourages screening, testing, and treatment and strengthens the capacity to monitor STD trends as part of a comprehensive STD prevention and health care program that is directed by trained health care professionals as a harm reduction agent presents a viable form of prevention to address the increasing STD diagnoses in the United States. In addition, it has the potential to save thousands of lives.

Critics of the harm reduction approach argue that these initiatives are a waste of taxpayer's money. *First*, many argue that the use of a harm reduction technique only encourages people to continue their destructive action. In the case of increasing accessibility and use of condoms, critics believe it will only lead to a higher STD infection rate because it will give some people a false sense of protection. Similarly, critics argue that these approaches lead people away from seeking testing and treatment because they now have a safety net of sorts for their risky behaviors. Some critics also believe that we would be wasting valuable money, when that money could be spent on prevention programs that are more ethical and socially acceptable. Proponents of the harm reduction theory point to the various successes of this approach. The needle and syringe exchange programs have decreased the HIV infection rate among IV drug users in the United States. The opioid substitution therapy (PST) or opioid replacement therapy (ORT) replaces illegal opioids, such as heroin, with a longer acting but less euphoric opioid such as methadone or buprenorphine under medical supervision. In addition, supervised injection sites provide sterile injection equipment, information about drugs and basic health care, treatment referrals, and access to health care professionals. All three examples show the efficacy of the harm reduction theory. Finally, to address these criticisms and to strengthen the arguments for this harm reduction approach, it must be determined whether broader access to the recommendations proposed would promote more good than harm, not only for the minority population but also for their associates and communities at large.

Ethically, the harm reduction theory can be grounded in the principle of proportionate reason. Proportionate reason refers to a specific value and its relation to all elements in action [58]. The specific value in following the recommendations to decrease the STD rate is to preserve human life by decreasing HIV infections, limiting other health care issues that result from STDs and encouraging responsible sexual behavior to vulnerable members of society. The harm, which may come about by trying to achieve this value, is the foreseen but unintended possibility that some may view this as condoning and even encouraging risky sexual behavior. The ethical question is whether the value of preserving human life outweighs the harm of the foreseen, but unintended, possibility of scandal and possible increased risky sexual behavior. To determine if a proper relationship exists between the specific value and other elements of the act, ethicist Richard McCormick, S.J. proposes three criteria for the establishment of proportionate reason as follows:

1. The means used will not cause more harm than necessary to achieve the value.

2. No less harmful way exists to protect the value.

3. The means used to achieve the value will not undermine it [59].

The application of McCormick's criteria to follow the recommendations in this paper supports the argument that there is a proportionate reason for not only allowing these recommendations but also for actively advocating for them. First, according to public health officials, without a "massive national public health effort" and increased funding and education, especially among the minority populations, the STD rate in the United States will continue to increase and more lives could be lost. According to public health officials, "Information, education and counseling can improve people's ability to recognize the symptoms of STIs and increase the likelihood that they will seek care and encourage sexual partners to do so; unfortunately, lack of public awareness, lack of training among health workers, and long-standing, widespread stigma around STIs remain barriers to greater and more effective use of these interventions" [27]. Unless we can address this epidemic now, the long-term effects can be devastating. According to Cleveland Clinic, more than 25 million sexually transmitted infections occur each year in the United States. Worldwide, we estimate 374 million sexually transmitted infections occur annually. According to CDC, 2.5 million cases of chlamydia, gonorrhea, and syphilis occurred in the United States in 2021. About half of these cases occur in people ages 15–24 years, and the majority are among minority populations [60]. We know STDs can lead to HIV infections and AIDS, can damage organs and the nervous system, and infect a developing fetus, increase ectopic pregnancies and pelvic inflammatory disease (PID). Unless we take drastic steps to decrease this STD rate, people's lives will continue to be in jeopardy. *Second*, at present, there are not any alternatives other than those we recommend for the at-risk population. It is true that other means of prevention exist such as abstinence, but according to health care authorities, abstinence is not realistic for many at-risk individuals. In the United States, 1 out of 8 HIV infected people out of the 1.2 million infected are unaware that they were infected and continue to infect others. Many of these infected and those with STDs are participating in risky sexual behavior. Advocating for the recommendations we propose such as correct and consistent condom use, safe and effective vaccines, money for new vaccine research, biomedical interventions that include voluntary medical male circumcision, microbicides, and partner treatment are the only methods that will help decrease the STD rates. This will entail educating our public health workers so that they can educate and counsel those who are most vulnerable. This human contact allows health care workers to form personal relationships with at-risk individuals and thus provides the opportunity to offer them appropriate health care, personal counseling, testing, and referrals to treatment centers. Various scientific studies have confirmed that intravenous drug users reduce risk-laden behaviors when pertinent information and services, such as counseling are made available, and especially when they are offered by peers who are members of the drug-using subcultures [61–63]. The same can be said for those participating in risky sexual behavior. Advocating for these recommendations to at-risk individuals by trained health care professionals has the potential not only to save human lives but also to foster human dignity and respect. *Third*, our recommendations do not undermine the value of human life. One can argue convincingly that the intention of making these recommendations available to at-risk individuals by trained health care professionals is to save human lives. This is a public health issue that must be addressed because innocent people are becoming infected and potentially these lives could be lost. It seems clear that there is a proportionate reason to put these recommendations into a national policy to be made available to all Americans using taxpayers' money. These recommendations contribute to the well-being of at-risk individuals and society because this tool has the potential to decrease the STD infection rate and ultimately save medical resources and human lives. It also offers those who are at risk the opportunity to realize that they are valued as individuals and, with the appropriate assistance, STD infections can be avoided, and the STD epidemic can be minimized. Therefore, it is ethically justified under the principle of proportionate reason to create a national policy with our proposed recommendations and to make these recommendations available to at-risk individuals at approved community-based organizations that are coordinated by health care professionals. Ethically, the greater good of those individuals at risk and the common good of society are advanced by financially supporting these recommendations in major cities in the United States.

6. Discussion and public health recommendations

With the causes of the recent surge in STI rates in mind, it is important to consider new and innovative methods to combat further increases. We herein propose initiatives that address current shortcomings from educational, accessibility, and financial perspectives.

6.1 Local partnerships

One barrier that prevents sexual education from resulting in behavioral changes is the relationship between the educator and the student. In schools, oftentimes, the teacher-student relationship may not be the best setting to survey this type of material. Additionally, many schools promote abstinence-based curricula, which do not reduce rates of self-reported STIs or pregnancy [64]. However, in settings that individuals trust, such as the barbershop, this barrier is removed, and education on this topic has the potential to be much more effective. In fact, a 2017 study of surveyed barbers found that the barbershops are embraced as a setting suitable for sexual education discussions given the close relationship between barbers and their clients [65]. As an example of this suitability, St. Louis began its "Fading Out HIV" initiative in 2015, as its Department of Health partnered with barbershops to administer free condoms and HIV/STI prevention education to clients of the shops [66]. The data from the city's HIV dashboard reveal that the rate of new HIV diagnoses in the city fell from 33 per 100,000 people in 2016 to 18 per 100,000 people in 2020 before rising again during the nationwide surge [67]. Similarly, in other locations, programs run through churches having increased mammograms and HIV testing among Black women [68]. While only a sample size of one city, this initiative has shown promise, and more importantly, has shown that trusted settings can be a launching pad for education, testing, and condom use.

6.2 TakeMeHome kits

In 2006, CDC announced a recommendation that anyone considered high-risk for HIV exposure should undergo HIV testing annually [69]. However, the stay-at-home orders brought on by the pandemic made this difficult to satisfy. Therefore, in March 2020, TakeMeHome HIV testing kits were distributed as a home care option for those disproportionately affected by HIV [58]. Marketing focused on gay, bisexual, and MSM communities [58]. A study by CDC revealed that 36% of kit users reported never having tested before, and over 50% last tested over a year prior to receiving the kit [58]. Encouragingly, over 10% of respondents who tested themselves accessed additional STI testing services, and 8% accessed pre-exposure prophylaxis (PrEP) treatment [58]. This intervention represents another potential method of improving access to testing and other services among at-risk communities.

6.3 Expedited partner therapy (EPT)

EPT is an approach to STI transmission reduction that involves clinicians prescribing STI treatment to partners of their patients without requiring clinical assessment of the partner [70]. This ideally allows partners to go pick up treatment prescriptions for the particular STI without going through the hassle of visiting a physician and obtaining the prescription himself or herself, which can be a barrier to treatment for some people. Additionally, some experts see this as a way to promote treatment in the age group of teenagers and young adults who may not know where to get treatment, may fear telling a parent about possible infection, or may not have the transportation to reach a provider [71]. A 2019 study simulating the effects of EPT over a 10-year period found that it has the potential to reduce population-level STI rates [72].

The legal situation surrounding this type of provider-patient relationship is an important aspect that cannot be overlooked when analyzing this as a possible solution to the surge in STI rates. Forty-six states currently have EPT as at least permissible by law, whereas in the other four, it is potentially permissible. Evidence suggests that having legislation explicitly supporting EPT could lead to decreased rates of STI, such as one 2018 study found to be true of chlamydia [73]. A CDC study found that among gonorrhea patients, 13% reported receipt of EPT in states in which EPT is supported by law, whereas only 5% of patients in states without supportive legislation received EPT [74]. Pennsylvania recently passed legislation to increase EPT freedoms for providers, which marks another possible remedy to the surging STI rates if more states follow suit.

6.4 Prophylactic doxycycline

Recent research suggests that a single dose of doxycycline within 72 hr. of exposure can significantly reduce the risk of bacterial STI transmission [75]. One study analyzing the effect of post-exposure prophylactic doxycycline treatment found that chlamydia and syphilis incidence dropped by 70 and 73%, respectively, whereas gonorrhea rates did not fall as much [76]. While CDC has yet to issue a formal recommendation for the use of doxycycline in this context, several other studies have since confirmed similar findings. In addition, some cities, such as San Francisco, are already offering this as a viable preventative option [77]. As with any antibiotic intervention, antimicrobial resistance is a concern with such an initiative should it become more widespread. However, experts have seen no evidence that single-dose doxycycline used in this context contributes to antibiotic resistance strains of bacterial STIs [66]. The current shortage in bicillin, the primary antibiotic used to fight syphilis infection, reinforces the importance of a prophylactic intervention so that patients avoid infection in the first place and are not left without antibiotics after the infection progresses [78]. Thus, based on available evidence, this appears to be a viable option to help combat the surge of STI transmission rates.

6.5 Further recommendations at the national level

1. *Federal Sexual Health Funding*: One of the more obvious contributions to the recent surge in STI rates is the decrease in funding for sexual health clinics nationally. According to the National Coalition of STD Directors, federal funding

for STD programs decreased from $168.5 million in 2003 to $152.5 million in 2022 [79]. This represents a 40% decrease when accounting for inflation [68]. In the United States, the recent mpox outbreak has shone a spotlight on this deficiency, and this must be remedied to truly reverse the trend of current STI rates.

2. *Promote the U.S. National Strategic Plan*: The WHO's position with regard to containing STIs worldwide is to support any country that adopts a concrete plan of action to prevent and treat STIs [80]. The Department of Health and Human Services released such a 5-year plan in 2020 for STIs control in the United States [81]. It is our recommendation that this become a focal point of government health and wellness initiatives nationwide to increase awareness of the issue.

3. *Primary STI Prevention and Care Expansion*: We also recommend that STI prevention be more intrinsic to regular primary care in the United States. This can include expanded condom availability in such settings and more education on prevention topics, among other tools.

4. *Strengthen Ability to Monitor STI Trends and Respond to Antimicrobial Resistance (AMR)*: We recommend that monitoring capabilities of STIs be strengthened to remain abreast with the latest effects that the infections are having on the population. This includes remaining vigilant about AMR versions of the pathogens and improving the country's ability to respond to the inevitable rises in AMR infections.

5. *Increase Research and Development for New Vaccines*: While such research is advanced for genital herpes and HIV, further efforts for chlamydia, gonorrhea, and syphilis are needed [69].

6. *Promote the Use of Other Biomedical Interventions*: We recommend the encouragement of other interventions, such as adult voluntary circumcision, microbicides, and pre/post-exposure prophylaxis to help mitigate the risk of transmission nationwide [69].

We understand that none of these interventions are single silver bullets that will fix the problem altogether and that there are many potential arguments against each of these initiatives. For example, the aforementioned "Fading Out HIV" initiative run in St. Louis barbershops has proven to be effective in certain communities, but one may argue that this effectiveness will not spread to other areas of the country where barbershops may not be a central or necessarily trusted part of the community. We recognize this concern and other concerns of this type, but we would counter that other institutions such as churches have also shown promise and that this recommendation of "Local Partnerships" can be extrapolated to whatever is the trusted and comfortable setting in a particular community or culture.

Expedited partner therapy is an initiative that has been particularly controversial given the apparent threat it poses to the traditional physician-patient relationship and the assumed dangers of giving medication to a patient that was never evaluated. Additionally, critics may argue that by providing EPT, the partner of the patient is missing out on a potential encounter with a physician that could reveal other health issues and counseling opportunities. However, we believe that the partner still has the ability to be evaluated despite the EPT if he or she so desires. In addition, the potential public health benefits of stemming the spread of infection at the level of two partners as quickly as possible outweighs many of the concerns noted by the critics of EPT.

We also acknowledge that perhaps the most popular critique of a prophylactic doxycycline pill after a sexual encounter is the risk of antimicrobial resistance. As mentioned previously, there has yet to be evidence supporting this idea that prophylactic doxycycline has this effect. Thus, it is our position that given the benefits currently posed by this intervention, we recommend its broad implementation. However, we acknowledge that upon possible future evidence, it increases the prevalence of antimicrobial resistance, we may alter our recommendation, as the benefits may no longer outweigh the risks of this intervention.

We also understand that many of the other proposed interventions require vast amounts of monetary investment and that large upfront costs for interventions that prove to have long-term benefits is not exactly a popular idea among politicians and taxpayers alike. However, as mentioned previously, it seems as though the government is valuing public health less and less as evidenced by the decrease in funding toward establishments such as STD clinics. However, we remain steadfast in our belief that given the long-term costs associated with untreated STIs, both medically and financially, increased investment in STI prevention is the most ethical and intelligent path forward from the U.S. government perspective.

7. Conclusions

Overall, with the rates of chlamydia, gonorrhea, and syphilis continuing to surge each year, there must be a change in methodology in the way that policymakers are facing the issue. This methodology shift should lean toward providing the youth with a comprehensive education and set of resources in order to be best prepared to have safe sexual relationships, rather than trying to limit the amount of education and resources that this group has access to. Through programs such as these, barriers to resources and education could be broken down; and with this, knowledge of health sexual encounters and resources for treatment, the transmission rates of these diseases could begin to fall; and it is imperative that they do.

Author details

Shrikanth Sampath[1], Mahvish Renzu[1], Peter Clark[2*], Joseph Kelly[3] and Daniel Disandro[4]

1 MD-PGY-2 Mercy Catholic Medical Center Darby, Pennsylvania, United States

2 John McShain Chain in Ethics Saint Joseph's University, Philadelphia, Pennsylvania, United States

3 Institute of Clinical Bioethics Saint Joseph's University Philadelphia, Pennsylvania, United States

4 Lewis Katz Medical School Temple University Philadelphia, Pennsylvania, United States

*Address all correspondence to: pclark@sju.edu

References

[1] Keller LH, Guttmacher Institute. Reducing STI Cases: Young People Deserve Better Sexual Health Information and Services. New York, NY, USA: Guttmacher Institute; 2022. Available from: https://www.guttmacher.org/gpr/2020/04/reducing-sti-cases-young-people-deserve-better-sexual-health-information-and-services

[2] Centers for Disease Control and Prevention. Sexually Transmitted Disease Surveillance, 2021. Atlanta, GA, USA: Centers for Disease Control and Prevention; 2023. Available from: https://www.cdc.gov/std/statistics/2021/default.html

[3] Hicks C, Clement M. Syphilis: Epidemiology, Pathophysiology, and Clinical Manifestations in Patients without HIV. Alphen aan den Rijn, Netherlands: UpToDate; 2023. Available from: https://www.uptodate.com/contents/syphilis-epidemiology-pathophysiology-and-clinical-manifestations-in-patients-without-hiv?search=Syphilis&source=search_result&selectedTitle=3~150&usage_type=default&display_rank=3

[4] Tampa M, Sarbu I, Matei C, Benea V, Georgescu SR. Brief history of syphilis. Journal of Medicine and Life. 2014;**7**(1):4-10. Epub 2014 Mar 25

[5] Clement ME, Okeke NL, Hicks CB. Treatment of syphilis: A systematic review. Journal of the American Medical Association. 2014;**312**(18):1905-1917. DOI: 10.1001/jama.2014.13259

[6] Centers for Disease Control and Prevention. Detailed Std Facts - Syphilis. Atlanta, GA, USA: Centers for Disease Control and Prevention; 2023. Available from: https://www.cdc.gov/std/syphilis/stdfact-syphilis-detailed.html

[7] Tuddenham S, Ghanem KG. Management of adult syphilis: Key questions to inform the 2021 Centers for Disease Control and Prevention sexually transmitted infections treatment guidelines. Clinical Infectious Diseases. 2022;**74**(Suppl. 2):S127-S133. DOI: 10.1093/cid/ciac060

[8] Centers for Disease Control and Prevention. CDC – Syphilis Treatment. Atlanta, GA, USA: Centers for Disease Control and Prevention; 2022. Available from: https://www.cdc.gov/std/syphilis/treatment.html

[9] Centers for Disease Control and Prevention. Syphilis during Pregnancy - STI Treatment Guidelines. Atlanta, GA, USA: Centers for Disease Control and Prevention; 2021. Available from: https://www.cdc.gov/std/treatment-guidelines/syphilis-pregnancy.html

[10] Centers for Disease Control and Prevention. Congenital Syphilis - STI Treatment Guidelines. Atlanta, GA, USA: Centers for Disease Control and Prevention; 2021. Available from: https://www.cdc.gov/std/treatment-guidelines/congenital-syphilis.html

[11] Cleveland Clinic. Gonorrhea: Causes, Symptoms, Treatment & Prevention. Cleveland, OH, USA: Cleveland Clinic; 2023. Available from: https://my.clevelandclinic.org/health/diseases/4217-gonorrhea

[12] Ghanem K. Clinical Manifestations and Diagnosis of *Neisseria Gonorrhoeae* Infection in Adults and Adolescents. Alphen aan den Rijn, Netherlands: UpToDate; 2023. Available from: https://www.uptodate.com/contents/clinical-manifestations-and-diagnosis-of-neisseria-gonorrhoeae-infection-in-adults-and-adolescen

ts?search=gonorrhea&source=search_result&selectedTitle=2~150&usage_type=default&display_rank=2

[13] US Preventive Services Task Force. Screening for chlamydia and gonorrhea: US preventive services task force recommendation statement. Journal of the American Medical Association. 2021;**326**(10):949-956. DOI: 10.1001/jama.2021.14081

[14] Unemo M, Seifert HS, Hook EW, et al. Gonorrhoea. Nature Reviews. Disease Primers. 2019;5:79. DOI: 10.1038/s41572-019-0128-6

[15] Centers for Disease Control and Prevention. Gonococcal Infections among Adolescents and Adults - STI Treatment Guidelines. Atlanta, GA, USA: Centers for Disease Control and Prevention; 2022. Available from: https://www.cdc.gov/std/treatment-guidelines/gonorrhea-adults.html

[16] Cleveland Clinic. Chlamydia: Causes, Symptoms, Treatment & Prevention. Cleveland, OH, USA: Cleveland Clinic; 2023. Available from: https://my.clevelandclinic.org/health/diseases/4023-chlamydia

[17] Centers for Disease Control and Prevention. Std Facts - Chlamydia. Atlanta, GA, USA: Centers for Disease Control and Prevention; 2022. Available from: https://www.cdc.gov/std/chlamydia/stdfact-chlamydia.html

[18] NHS Choices. Chlamydia Fact Sheet. London, UK: NHS; 2021. Available from: https://www.nhs.uk/conditions/chlamydia/symptoms/

[19] Mohseni M, Sung S, Takov V. Chlamydia. Treasure Island (FL): StatPearls Publishing; 2023. Available from: https://www.ncbi.nlm.nih.gov/books/NBK537286/

[20] Meyer T. Diagnostic procedures to detect *C. trachomatis* infections. Microorganisms. 2016;**4**(3):25. DOI: 10.3390/microorganisms4030025

[21] Centers for Disease Control and Prevention. Chlamydial Infections - STI Treatment Guidelines. Atlanta, GA, USA: Centers for Disease Control and Prevention; 2021. Available from: https://www.cdc.gov/std/treatment-guidelines/chlamydia.html

[22] Centers for Disease Control and Prevention, "STD Facts - Syphilis & MSM." Atlanta, GA, USA: Centers for Disease Control and Prevention; 11 Apr 2023. Available from: https://www.cdc.gov/std/syphilis/stdfact-msm-syphilis.html

[23] Tsuboi M, Evans J, Davies EP, Rowley J, Korenromp EL, Clayton T, et al. Prevalence of syphilis among men who have sex with men: A global systematic review and meta-analysis from 2000-20. The Lancet Global Health. 2021;**9**(8):e1110-e1118. DOI: 10.1016/S2214-109X(21)00221-7. Epub 2021 Jul 8

[24] Solomon MM, Mayer KH. Evolution of the syphilis epidemic among men who have sex with men. Sexual Health. 2015;**12**(2):96-102. DOI: 10.1071/SH14173

[25] Centers for Disease Control and Prevention. Primary Prevention Methods. Atlanta, GA, USA: Centers for Disease Control and Prevention; 2023. Available from: https://www.cdc.gov/std/treatment-guidelines/clinical-primary.html#CautionsForDoxyPEP

[26] Centers for Disease Control and Prevention. STD Health Equity. Atlanta, GA, USA: Centers for Disease Control and Prevention; 2020. Available from: https://www.cdc.gov/std/health-disparities/default.html

[27] World Health Organization, "Sexually Transmitted Infections (Stis)."

Geneva, Switzerland: World Health Organization; 2023. Available from: www.who.int/news-room/fact-sheets/detail/sexually-transmitted-infections-(stis). [Accessed: May 10, 2023]

[28] Office of Infectious Disease and HIV/AIDS Policy (OIDP). Sexually Transmitted Infections (Stis). Washington, DC, USA: OIDP; 2022, HHS.Gov, Available from: www.hhs.gov/programs/topic-sites/sexually-transmitted-infections/index.html

[29] Institute of Medicine (US) Committee on Prevention and Control of Sexually Transmitted Diseases; Eng TR, Butler WT, editors. The Hidden Epidemic: Confronting Sexually Transmitted Diseases. Washington (DC): National Academies Press (US); 1997. 2, the neglected health and economic impact of STDs. Available from: https://www.ncbi.nlm.nih.gov/books/NBK232938/

[30] Tsevat DG, Wiesenfeld HC, Parks C, Peipert JF. Sexually transmitted diseases and infertility. American Journal of Obstetrics and Gynecology. 2017;**216**(1):1-9. DOI: 10.1016/j.ajog.2016.08.008

[31] Workowski KA, Berman SM. Centers for Disease Control and Prevention sexually transmitted disease treatment guidelines. Atlanta, GA, USA: Clinical Infectious Diseases. 2011;**53**(suppl_3):S59-S63. DOI: 10.1093/cid/cir694

[32] Centers for Disease Control and Prevention. Infertility & Stds - STD Information from CDC. Atlanta, GA, USA: Centers for Disease Control and Prevention; 2023. Available from: www.cdc.gov/std/infertility/default.html#:~:text=Untreated%2C%20about%2010%2D15%25,which%20can%20lead%20to%20infertility

[33] Ness RB, Markovic N, Carlson CL, Coughlin MT. Do men become infertile after having sexually transmitted urethritis? An epidemiologic examination. Fertility and Sterility. 1997;**68**(2):205-213. DOI: 10.1016/s0015-0282(97)81502-6

[34] Sobinoff AP, Dando SJ, Redgrove KA, Sutherland JM, Stanger SJ, Armitage CW, et al. Chlamydia muridarum infection-induced destruction of male germ cells and sertoli cells is partially prevented by chlamydia major outer membrane protein-specific immune CD4 cells. Biology of Reproduction. 2015;**92**(1):27. DOI: 10.1095/biolreprod.114.124180. Epub 2014 Dec 3

[35] World Health Organization. Prevalence and Incidence of Selected Sexually Transmitted Infections, *Chlamydia trachomatis*, *Neisseria gonorrhoeae*, Syphilis and Trichomonas Vaginalis: Methods and Results Used by WHO to Generate 2005 Estimates. Geneva, Switzerland: World Health Organization; 2011. Available from: https://apps.who.int/iris/handle/10665/44735

[36] Oakeshott P, Kerry S, Aghaizu A, Atherton H, Hay S, Taylor-Robinson D, et al. Randomised controlled trial of screening for *Chlamydia trachomatis* to prevent pelvic inflammatory disease: The POPI (prevention of pelvic infection) trial. BMJ. 2010;**340**:c1642. DOI: 10.1136/bmj.c1642

[37] Brunham RC, Gottlieb SL, Paavonen J. Pelvic inflammatory disease. The New England Journal of Medicine. 2015;**372**(21):2039-2048. DOI: 10.1056/NEJMra1411426

[38] Chesson HW, Mayaud P, Aral SO. Sexually transmitted infections: Impact and cost-effectiveness of prevention. In: Holmes KK, Bertozzi S, Bloom BR, et al., editors. Major Infectious Diseases. 3rd ed. Washington (DC): The International Bank for Reconstruction

and Development/The World Bank; 2017. Chapter 10. Available from: https://www.ncbi.nlm.nih.gov/books/NBK525195/. DOI: 10.1596/978-1-4648-0524-0_ch10

[39] Chin-Hong P et al. STD Epidemic in US Carries Staggering Human, Economic Costs. Thorofare, NJ, USA: Healio; 2017. Available from: www.healio.com/news/infectious-disease/20170208/std-epidemic-in-us-carries-staggering-human-economic-costs

[40] Craig-Kuhn MC, Schmidt N, Lederer A, Gomes G, Watson S, Scott G Jr, et al. Sex education and STI fatalism, testing and infection among young African American men who have sex with women. Sex Education. 2021;**21**(4):404-416. DOI: 10.1080/14681811.2020.1809369. Epub 2020 Sep 9

[41] Centers for Disease Control and Prevention. HIV/STD Prevention at a Glance. Atlanta, GA, USA: Centers for Disease Control and Prevention; 2020. Available from: www.cdc.gov/healthyyouth/about/hivstd_prevention.html

[42] Centers for Disease Control and Prevention. Detailed Std Facts - HIV/AIDS & Stds. Atlanta, GA, USA: Centers for Disease Control and Prevention; 2023. Available from: www.cdc.gov/std/hiv/stdfact-std-hiv-detailed.html

[43] Myhre J, Sifris D. 3 Surprising Ways that Stds Increase HIV Risk. New York, NY, USA: Verywell Health; 2022. Available from: www.verywellhealth.com/stds-increase-hiv-risk-49603

[44] Lynn WA, Lightman S. Syphilis and HIV: A dangerous combination. The Lancet Infectious Diseases. 2004;**4**(7):456-466, ISSN 1473-3099. DOI: 10.1016/S1473-3099(04)01061-8

[45] Fan L, Aiping Y, Zhang D, Wang Z, Ma P. Consequences of HIV/syphilis co-infection on HIV viral load and immune response to antiretroviral therapy. Infection and Drug Resistance. 2021;**14**:2851-2862. DOI: 10.2147/IDR.S320648

[46] Wu MY, Gong HZ, Hu KR, et al. Effect of syphilis infection on HIV acquisition: A systematic review and meta-analysis. Sexually Transmitted Infections. 2021;**97**:525-533

[47] Kalichman SC, Pellowski J. Turner C prevalence of sexually transmitted co-infections in people living with HIV/AIDS: Systematic review with implications for using HIV treatments for prevention. Sexually Transmitted Infections. 2011;**87**:183-190

[48] Ren M, Dashwood T, Walmsley S. The intersection of HIV and syphilis: Update on the key considerations in testing and management. Current HIV/AIDS Reports. 2021;**18**:280-288. DOI: 10.1007/s11904-021-00564-z

[49] World Health Organization. Four Curable Sexually Transmitted Infections - all you Need to Know. Geneva, Switzerland: World Health Organization; 2019. Available from: www.who.int/news-room/feature-stories/detail/four-curable-sexually-transmitted-infections---all-you-need-to-know [Accessed: May 14, 2023]

[50] World Health Organization. Trachoma. Geneva, Switzerland: World Health Organization; 2022. Available from: www.who.int/news-room/fact-sheets/detail/trachoma#:~:text=Trachoma%20is%20a%20disease%20of,Blindness%20from%20trachoma%20is%20irreversible [Accessed: May 14, 2023]

[51] Centers for Disease Control and Prevention, "New Data Suggest Stds Continued to Increase during First Year of the COVID-19 Pandemic." Atlanta, GA, USA: Centers for Disease Control and

Prevention; 2022. Available from: https://www.cdc.gov/media/releases/2022/p0412-STD-Increase.html#:~:text=The%20data%20provide%20the%20clearest,%2C%20respectively%2C%20compared%20to%202019

[52] "Pittsburgh Post-Gazette: Poor Health." Barriers to Health Care for Low-Income America. Available from: https://newsinteractive.post-gazette.com/longform/stories/poorhealth/1/

[53] Haley DF, Edmonds A, Belenky N, Hickson DA, Ramirez C, Wingood GM, et al. Neighborhood health care access and sexually transmitted infections among women in the southern United States: A cross-sectional multilevel analysis. Sexually Transmitted Diseases. 2018;**45**(1):19-24. DOI: 10.1097/OLQ.0000000000000685

[54] Centers for Disease Control and Prevention. U.S. STI Epidemic Showed No Signs of Slowing in 2021-Cases Continued to Escalate. Atlanta, GA, USA: CDC; 2023

[55] Harm Reduction Coalition. Principles of Harm Reduction. New York, NY, USA: Harm Reduction Coalition; 2014. Available from: http://harmreduction.org/about-us/principles-of-harm-reduction/

[56] Hawk M, Coulter R, Egan J, Fisk S, Friedman R, Tula M, et al. Harm reduction principles for healthcare settings. Harm Reduction Journal. 2017;**14**:70. DOI: 10.1186/s12954-017-0196-4

[57] Marlatt A, Witkiewitz K. Update on harm-reduction policy and intervention research. Annual Review of Clinical Psychology. 2010;**6**:591-606

[58] Walter J. Proportionate reason and its three levels of inquiry: Structuring the ongoing debate. Louvain Studies. 1984;**10**:32

[59] McCormick R. McCormick's Criteria for Proportionate Reason First Appeared in Ambiguity In Moral Choice. Milwaukee, WI: Marquette University Press; 1973. He later reworked the criteria in response to criticism. His revised criteria can be found in Doing Evil To Achieve Good, eds. Richard McCormick and Paul Ramsey (Chicago, IL.: Loyola University Press, 1978)

[60] Cleveland Clinic. Sexually Transmitted Infections. Cleveland, OH, USA: Cleveland Clinic; 2023. Available from: http://my.clevelandclinic.org/health/disease/9138-sexually-tranbsmitted-diseases-infections-stds-stis

[61] American Medical Association's Council On Scientific Affairs: 10. See also, Booth R, Wiebel W. Effectiveness of reducing needle-related risks for HIV through indigenous outreach to injection drug users. American Journal of Addictions. 1992;**1**:277-287

[62] Neaigus A, Sufian M, Friedman SR, et al. Efforts of outreach intervention on risk reduction among intravenous drug users. AIDS Education Prevention. 1990;**2**:253-271

[63] Watters J, Downing M, Case P, et al. AIDS prevention for intravenous drug users in the community: Street based education and risk behavior. American Journal of Community Psychology. 1990;**18**:587-596

[64] Mason-Jones AJ, Sinclair D, Mathews C, Kagee A, Hillman A, Lombard C. School-based interventions for preventing HIV, sexually transmitted infections, and pregnancy in adolescents. Cochrane Database of Systematic Reviews. 2016;**2016**(11):CD006417. DOI: 10.1002/14651858.cd006417.pub3

[65] Randolph SD, Pleasants T, Gonzalez-Guarda RM. Barber-led sexual health education intervention for black male adolescents and their fathers. Public Health Nursing. 2017;**34**(6):555-560. DOI: 10.1111/phn.12350

[66] City of St. Louis. City of St. Louis Department of Health Partners with Barbers and Hairstylists to "Fade out" Sexually Transmitted Infections. St. Louis, MO, USA: City of St. Louis. Stlouis-mo.gov. Available from: https://www.stlouis-mo.gov/government/departments/health/news/doh-partners-with-barbers-and-hairstylists-to-fade-out-stis.cfm; 2015 [Accessed: April 22, 2023]

[67] City of St. Louis. Fast-Track Cities HIV Data. St. Louis, MO, USA: City of St. Louis. Stlouis-mo.gov. Available from: https://www.stlouis-mo.gov/hiv/data/totals.cfm; 2021 [Accessed: April 22, 2023]

[68] Tingley K. Why Are Sexually Transmitted Infections Surging? New York, NY, USA: The New York Times; Available from https://www.nytimes.com/2022/05/17/magazine/sexually-transmitted-infections-surging.html; 2022 [Accessed: April 22, 2023]

[69] Hecht J, Sanchez T, Sullivan PS, DiNenno EA, Cramer N, Delaney KP. Increasing access to HIV testing through direct-to-consumer HIV self-test distribution—United States, March 31, 2020–March 30, 2021. MMWR. Morbidity and Mortality Weekly Report. 2021;**70**:1322-1325. DOI: 10.15585/mmwr.mm7038a2

[70] Centers for Disease Control and Prevention. Legal Status of Expedited Partner Therapy (EPT). Atlanta, GA, USA: Centers for Disease Control and Prevention. Available from: https://www.cdc.gov/std/ept/legal/default.html; 2021 [Accessed: April 22, 2023]

[71] Laughlin J. A New Pa. Law Is Giving Doctors Greater Freedom to Treat People with Sexually Transmitted Diseases. Philadelphia, PA, USA: The Philadelphia Inquirer. Available from: https://www.inquirer.com/health/sexually-transmitted-infection-gonorrhea-chlamydia-pennsylvania-treatment-20230203.html; 2023 [Accessed: April 22, 2023]

[72] Weiss KM, Jones JS, Katz DA, Gift TL, Bernstein K, Workowski K, et al. Epidemiological impact of expedited partner therapy for men who have sex with men: A modeling study. Sexually Transmitted Diseases. 2019;**46**(11):697-705. DOI: 10.1097/OLQ.0000000000001058

[73] Mmeje O, Wallet S, Kolenic G, Bell J. Impact of expedited partner therapy (EPT) implementation on chlamydia incidence in the USA. Sexually Transmitted Infections. 2017;**94**(7):545-547. DOI: 10.1136/sextrans-2016-052887

[74] Cramer R, Leichliter JS, Stenger MR, Loosier PS, Slive L. The legal aspects of expedited partner therapy practice. Sexually Transmitted Diseases. 2013;**40**(8):657-662. DOI: 10.1097/01.olq.0000431358.18959.d4

[75] Mandavilli A. These Morning-after Pills May Prevent STDs, Researchers Say. New York, NY, USA: The New York Times. Available from: https://www.nytimes.com/2023/03/09/health/syphilis-chlamydia-gonorrhea-doxycycline.html; 2023. [Accessed: April 22, 2023]

[76] Molina JM, Charreau I, Chidiac C, Pialoux G, Cua E, Delaugerre C, et al. Post-exposure prophylaxis with doxycycline to prevent sexually

transmitted infections in men who have sex with men: An open-label randomised substudy of the ANRS IPERGAY trial. The Lancet. Infectious Diseases. 2018;**18**(3):308-317. DOI: 10.1016/S1473-3099(17)30725-9

[77] Department of Public Health, City & County of San Francisco. Doxy-PEP. San Francisco, CA, USA: San Francisco City Clinic. Available from: https://www.sfcityclinic.org/services/sti-and-hiv-prevention/doxy-pep; n.d. [Accessed: April 22, 2023]

[78] Ryan B. Antibiotic Shortage Could Worsen Syphilis Epidemic. New York, NY, USA: The New York Times; 2023. Available from: https://www.nytimes.com/2023/07/07/health/syphilis-epidemic-antibiotic-shortage-pfizer.html. [Accessed: July 18, 2023]

[79] Steenhuysen J, Rigby J. Analysis: Years of Neglect Leaves Sexual Health Clinics Ill-Prepared for Monkeypox. Toronto, ON, Canada: Reuters. Available from: https://www.reuters.com/business/healthcare-pharmaceuticals/years-neglect-leaves-sexual-health-clinics-ill-prepared-monkeypox-2022-07-18/#:~:text=Federal%20funding%20for%20STD%20programs,inflation%2C%20according%20to%20the%20NCSD; 2022. [Accessed: April 22, 2023]

[80] World Health Organization. Sexually Transmitted Infections (STIs). Geneva, Switzerland: World Health Organization; 2022. Available from: https://www.who.int/news-room/fact-sheets/details/sexually-transmitted-infections-(sti

[81] U.S. Department of Health and Human Services. Sexually Transmitted Infections National Strategic Plan for the United States: 2021-2025. Washington, DC: U.S. Department of Health and Human Services; 2020

Chapter 10

Procedural, Substantive, and By-Design Approach toward a Third Stage of Bioethics

Salvador Ribas Ribas

Abstract

The central idea of this paper is that in bioethics there are two types of discourses or approaches, one procedural and the other one substantive or content approach. The first one seems to be predominant because it responds better to the demand in contemporary times by offering procedures, rules, and guidelines to help healthcare professionals to find solutions to ethical issues, rather than the second one, which is focused on the trait of characters, attitudes, and the moral content. Since the digital era started, data as moral content and systems have become the most valuable resource. This has been manifested in multiple areas such as social network, business, and politics, among others. In medicine, the potential impact of novel technologies based on data like artificial intelligence and machine learning, among others, may bring preventive, diagnostic, and therapeutic benefits for patients as well as result in potential issues, and the majority are still unknown. In order to guarantee respect to the new moral content, and compliance with bioethics principles within procedures and systems in the digital era a third approach is required: bioethics by-design.

Keywords: bioethics, principles, procedures, content, substantive, data, digital technologies, by-design

1. Introduction

Ethics and medicine share the goal of finding solutions to issues, and the difference between the two disciplines is that while the first deals with those conflicts that are related to human's values, interests, or preferences, the second deals with health problems. Like ethics and medicine, one of the main objectives pursued by bioethics has been to help healthcare professionals to resolve ethical issues that appear in their daily clinical practice.

Daniel Buchanan argued that bioethics has three main functions: identifying and defining existing ethical conflicts; providing systems or methods to think about new, emerging ethical conflicts in the field of medicine; and helping scientists and physicians to make decisions [1]. More than 50 years after Buchanan's article was published, clear evidence exists that systems, methods, and procedures are the predominant key elements to support healthcare professionals in benefitting patients and the clinical research. Therefore, there is a greater interest and demand for procedures, leaving aside questions related to the content and moral foundation of the decisions, as stated by N. Kass years ago [2].

Interest toward the decision-making procedures in solving ethical conflicts has resulted in a bioethics concept defined by Pincoffs as quandary ethics [3]. This focuses on finding solutions to conflicts by asking questions such as "What should I do?" or "What is correct?," leading to a significant reductionism: being moral simply means that you should be responsible for complying with a norm or an ethical principle. *Quandary ethics* puts more emphasis on the rules and procedures, and less on the content, and increasingly it seems that bioethics is acquiring the same classification as quandary ethics. This reductionism in bioethics is evident under the procedural approach of bioethics or principialism. As stated by Mark Siegler in 1985: "The central question that has occupied a generation of American bioethicists has been this: *Procedurally*, where should decision-making power reside — with the physician or with the patient? A quite different question, and one that has been of much greater concern to clinicians as ethicists, is this: What is the right and the good decision for this particular patient in these clinical circumstances? In bioethics literature, however, ideas of right and good decisions have often been subordinated to *procedural standards*" [4]. This is what some classify as reductionism, to reduce bioethics under the procedural approach of bioethics or principialism.

Indeed, we are faced with two ways of understanding bioethics, the procedural approach and the content or substantive approach.

2. Procedural bioethics and content or substantive bioethics

In the second half of the twentieth century, the practice of medicine entered a stage where mistrust between physicians and patients became the predominant note. It was then that codes and declarations were formulated to achieve greater regulation of clinical research in humans to protect patients' rights, like the Nuremberg Code (1947) or the Helsinki Declaration (1964).

Between the sixties and eighties, due to new technological advances applied in medicine for diagnosis and treatments, serious and unexpected ethical conflicts took place in the United States related to the practice of medicine. For example, the case in Seattle, and for the Karen Ann Quinlan case, see [5]. It was then that the first bioethics centers were created: the Institute of Society, Ethics and the Life Sciences, Hastings Center (1969), and the Joseph and Rose Kennedy Institute of Ethics for the Study of Human Reproduction and Bioethics (1971) in North America, and the Institut Borja de Bioètica (1975) in Europe. At this time, the Belmont Report was published, proposing three fundamental ethical principles that aimed to protect patients and justify actions in clinical research: the principle of autonomy, the principle of beneficence, and the principle of justice [6]. During the eighties, following this publication, the bioethical discourse was mainly built on formulating ethical principles to act as a basis for medical practice and clinical research.

Principles of Biomedical Ethics (1979) [7], Theory of Medical Ethics (1981) [8], and The Foundations of Bioethics (1986) [9] include the common feature to defend principles and procedures to solve ethical conflicts in the clinical field, in what at the bioethics discipline we understand as principlism. However, the most established procedural approach was the one defended by Beauchamp and Childress. The objective of their theory is to offer a reference framework for moral discernment and decision making and demonstrate how ethical theory can help to solve ethical issues in healthcare. They argue that not all areas of morality can be introduced within the theory of virtue's framework and language without supposing to lose basic moral protection. Moral judgment based on virtue ethics tends to be less important than rights and procedures. This may happen in relationships between strangers, for example, when a patient meets their physician for the first time. Therefore, a reference moral framework was proposed, providing four ethical principles that facilitate a common moral language in the patient-physician relationship: the principles of autonomy, non-maleficence, beneficence, and justice.

Robert M. Veatch, influenced by John Rawls' contractual theory, justified also a procedural bioethical theory on the basis of a triple contract [10]. In the face of ethical issues, the theory proposes a mixed strategy that includes a hierarchical or lexicographical order and weighting among several ethical principles. The lexicographical order is a serial order between principles that avoids having to level them, as there are those that have absolute value and remain without exception. These principles are a result of different contracts between people, and we add "between content," who seek to find a moral foundation for human actions within the same society or moral community.

Another example of procedural approach is the one proposed by H. Tristram Engelhardt based on the assumption that a contemporary society is constituted by relationships between moral strangers—between people who do not share the same morality (not share the same content)—and procedural bioethics allows coexistence between moral strangers as well as the creation of a moral community with a certain consensus among all. In other words, there are two moral discourses: the one between moral friends (the ones who are sharing content) and the one between moral strangers [9]. To have a moral discourse accepted by all parties, it is necessary to reach an agreement between moral strangers. This agreement or moral consensus may be achieved with two principles of the first order: the principle of permission, also called the principle of moral authority, and the principle of beneficence.

Theories by Beauchamp, Childress, Veatch, and Engelhardt are clear examples of what we may call the procedural approach in bioethics: those focused on rules and principles governed by procedures, rather than on content. We can reduce such theories as follows: The correct human act should be the result of acting according to a procedure.

The concept of "virtue" held a special relevance in the philosophy of ancient Greece, of the Middle Ages, and later in the Scottish Sentimental School. However, interest then dropped so low that it has been described as a "neglected topic" [11], a concept forgotten by contemporary moral philosophy. It was not until 1958 when Elizabeth Anscombe wrote her article "Modern Moral Philosophy" [12] that new articles and books began to appear in which virtue returned to occupy the center of attention of ethical theories. After Anscombe's article, several speeches were made that opposed the pre-eminence of concepts such as "moral duty" and "norm," and, in general, those deontological theories that suffered from excessive formality. This criticism of defining the moral act as a fulfillment of a duty or moral rule, or with the calculation of consequences, gave rise to the rebirth of aretaic ethics theories. In such theories, the intention and will of humans precede any action, and hence, the pre-eminence of character and its content are the foundation of moral discernment, instead of a set of principles or rules. Thus, a good act is not the result of acting according to a rule or principle, or after calculating that the benefits of an action outweigh its risks, or in accordance with a procedure. Instead, it is the result of acting on a virtue to achieve the good, requiring prior knowledge about what is good, rather than what is right. As Rosemarie Hursthouse summarizes, the ethics of virtue is the one centered on the agent and considers aretaic concepts such as "good" or "virtue," and not others, such as "right," "duty," and "obligation." In addition, it rejects the idea that ethics can encode rules or principles that guide actions [13].

The same occurred in bioethics: Concepts like virtue and moral content were forgotten due to a preference for principles and procedures. Despite the danger of forgetting bioethics of content, there have been several authors who have focused their bioethics theories on the aretaic approach [14, 15].

One of the main bioethics theories focused on content and aretaic concepts is the moral philosophy of medicine defended by Edmund D. Pellegrino and David Thomasma: a theory based on phenomenology of medicine and research on medical phenomena and its own content, such as the nature of health and disease. For Pellegrino, the ethics of medicine based on principles has certain shortcomings: "It leaves an inferential gap between principles and their application in concrete clinical cases. It is not convincing to physicians, because it is derived from philosophies external to medicine" [16]. Therefore, a philosophy of medicine is needed to provide the basis to define what good medicine is, content, and how duties, obligations, and rules, so procedures, should be derived from the content.

Medicine is not just a theoretical science but also a practice and a moral activity, like each human activity, since actions must be good as well as correct and right. In the medical field, we always find uncertainty, and the good of the patient depends, ultimately, on the nature (content) of each patient. In fact, both in diagnosis and in treatment, this uncertainty is inevitable, since there is no direct connection between medical science and the patient, between theoretical knowledge and the nature of each patient, between procedures or good practices and the patient. The uncertainty is also felt by the physician and investigators as they may not always have full evidence, full content, and all data about the best treatment, and not all of them are equally capable of making the best decision or best incisions. That's why neither a principle nor a procedure will help the physician or investigator to make the best decision or perform the incision, but a practical virtue to combat the medicine and clinical research uncertainty. As Pellegrino stated: "this irreducibility of the character of the moral agent, the physician in medical ethics, is a fact, regardless of the model of ethical reasoning one elects -principle- or rule-based, duty-based, casuistic, situational, emotivist, egoistic, intuitionist, and so on. In every ethical theory there comes a moment of opportunity, the use of the theory by a particular person in a particular circumstance. In that moment, the virtues will make the difference, making a good theory better in ameliorating the harm of erroneous theories" [15]. Thus, the content bioethics approach is focused on the content, on the actual interaction between the physician and the patient, rather than the formulation of procedures. A good act is the result of acting according to knowledge about what is good rather than following a principle, norm, rule, or procedure.

2.1 Procedural and content bioethics, toward a complementary approach

Despite the existence of multiple bioethical theories focused on virtue and content, such as the ethics of virtue by Pellegrino and Thomasma, the casuistic of Albert Jonsen [17], R. Tong's feminist approach [18], or the pragmatism defended by J.J. Fins and G. McGee [19], there is greater interest and need in procedural approaches to address the persistent emergence of ethical conflicts in healthcare and clinical research. The pre-eminence of procedural discourses is evident in clinical research: Decisions in research are subordinated to the protocol and study procedures. The essential trait of the procedural bioethical approach is that it focuses on the formulation of procedures that help solve ethical conflicts in clinical practice while respecting the principles and rules. Thus, the right action is carried out according to the procedure, and the ultimate responsibility depends on the grade of compliance to the procedure; the responsibility does not fall on the person but on rules and procedures. That is, there are not good or bad decisions, but rather better or worse procedures; there are not human errors, but technical issues. However, as Frankena states, "principles without traits are impotent and traits without principles are blind" [20], and the same could be said for the procedural bioethical approach and the content approach, as both are complementary. In that sense, Beauchamp and Childress also agree to incorporate virtues and principles into the same discourse; for them, "a moral philosophy is simply more complete if the virtues are integrated with principles. We have grounds to declare virtue theory and principlism partners rather than competitors" [21].

As stated by E. Pellegrino, bioethics principles help create a common discourse between healthcare professionals by facilitating a *lingua franca* [22] and an interdisciplinary dialog; however, procedures also need content because, by themselves, they do not exhaust the moral complexity of medicine.

In summary, a disjunction between substantive or content and procedural approach is not recommended. Virtue discourse is what confers moral content to the procedural discourse, overcoming any emptiness of the principle, or as Leo R. Kass called it, its "procedural ingenuity" [23]. The first is the set of bioethical theories giving prominence to virtue and placing greater interest toward the questions of foundation and content rather than the formulation of principles and procedures. The second is the one defended by those bioethical theories that, given the presence of ethical conflicts, facilitate decision-making processes to help find solutions and correct ways to act through the formulation of principles or procedures. Rather than rivals, the approaches should be complementary, as the first overcomes any procedural ingenuity, while virtue ethics provides moral content, substantive approach, principlism, and the procedural approach provides normativity.

2.2 Procedural and substantive bioethics in the physician-patient relationship

Since the middle of the twentieth century, the way of understanding the physician-patient relationship has been changing due to the socialization of medicine, its specialization, and the continuous technological advances. Since then, the bioethical discourse has tried to describe the physician-patient relationship with different models or metaphors: the paternalistic or autonomy model, the contract, alliance, or negotiation model, and the mutual participation model, among others (For example, see [24–32]).

In the physician-patient relationship, the distinction between procedural and content, substantive, or aretaic discourse is reflected more specifically in the distinction that Pellegrino and Thomasma establish between the contractual model and the fiduciary model. In the first one, the relationship is supported by a contract and is based on the assumption that a physician and a patient are moral strangers. This would be the model in accordance with the procedural proposals of Veatch and Engelhardt, who from a contractual model assume that a physician and a patient hardly share the same system of moral values. In the second model, the relationship is established based on mutual trust, assuming that there is some friendship between the physician and the patient, hence Pellegrino's critique: "autonomy-driven models of the doctor-patient relationship make the relationship largely instrumental and procedural. They are legalistic in spirit, and the ethics they engender is one minimal personal commitment and trust. Indeed, they are more based on distrust than trust" [22].

Indeed, Pellegrino and Thomasma maintain that there is no need for a contract or procedure to guarantee that the physician will act to achieve the good of the patient, something already implicit in the therapeutic relationship. They themselves recognize that, despite the fact that trust between a physician and a patient is replaced by a procedure in the contractual model, this does not mean that trust continues to be an essential element in the physician-patient relationship. Not only do they claim that contractual models replace friendship with a contract, but also, they can create a climate of mistrust between physicians and patients.

As summary, we can affirm there is no single model of the physician-patient relationship that contemplates all the variability of clinical practice as there is no single approach in bioethics. Moreover, in current times, both contractual elements, like informed consent procedures, protocol procedures, and good clinical practices, and fiduciary elements, like trust, attitude, and good intentions, are living together with.

2.2.1 Procedural and substantive bioethics approach in the field of ethics committees

The presence of ethics committees in hospitals began between the 60s and 70s in the United States, due to the emergence of new ethical issues as a result of scientific and technical advances in medicine. One of the first committees was the one created in Seattle, in 1961, with the purpose of deciding which patients would be given access or not to a new dialysis treatment, given the large number of patients and the scarcity of resources. Another committee was the Optimum Care Committee, which was created at the Massachusetts General Hospital in 1974 to help physicians to deal with ethical conflicts that arise in borderline situations, such as cardiopulmonary resuscitation [33]. Two years later, following the Quinlan case, the New Jersey Supreme Court recommended that hospitals have ethics committees [34]. Committees in Seattle, Massachusetts, and New Jersey were created on an *ad hoc* basis to address specific ethical issues that have arisen in areas of healthcare. It was not until the late 1980s that different US organizations expressed the need to create ethics committees in hospitals, as in 1983 the President's Commission for the Study of Ethical Problems in Medicine and Biomedical and Behavioral Research [35], the American Hospital Association [36], and the American Medical Association [37], who recommended the creation of ethics committees in hospitals to review and consult those cases in which medical decisions directly affected the life of a person. As the results of some surveys carried out on both healthcare professionals and patients in various centers in the US show, ethics committees in hospitals are necessary, and their presence is also generally valued as positive (For example, see [38–40]).

Years ago, as part of our initial research, an empirical study on healthcare ethics committees, the CEA-CAT study, was conducted in Catalonia with two main objectives: to know their structure and complete a self-assessment, and to find out what is more relevant for their members, such questions regarding procedures or questions regarding to the content of bioethics. The results showed that there was indeed a slight preeminence of procedural bioethical discourse with two main indicators: the recognition by the ethics committees themselves of being in greater possession of procedural skills rather than skills related to ethical content and interpersonal skills, and secondly, almost all committees have some kind of decision-making procedure [41].

However, in favor of the aretaic or content discourse, the same members that acknowledge having more procedural skills have the opinion that skills related to ethical content and interpersonal skills, like the attitude and character, are more important than procedural ones. In order words, one is more competent as more interest and intention is possessing, which reinforces the importance of the aretaic or substantive discourse to the detriment of the procedural one: that someone has an interest and the good redounds in their competence.

We demonstrated that there was a greater presence of procedural aspects: Almost all healthcare ethics committees have a decision-making process, and committee members are more in possession with procedural skills rather than content or interpersonal skills. However, the fact that there is a greater predominance of procedural aspects does not diminish the importance of aretaic or content aspects. Despite the indications that indicate a preference for procedural aspects, there is no evidence of theoretical forgetfulness of those aspects that have to do with the content and virtues. Thus, we can conclude there is a good coexistence between procedural and content or substantive aspects in the field of ethics committees also.

3. Digital health and data, toward a new era

Since the digital era started, there is no doubt that data and metadata have become the most valuable resource, as published in The Economist: "The world's most valuable resource is no longer oil, but data" [42]. This has been manifested in social networks, communication, business, education, and politics, among other fields and disciplines.

In medicine and clinical research, data must be reliable, robust, and credible in benefit to the patient and guarantee the best treatment, and multiple guidelines, regulations, and procedures have been established to achieve this goal, as for example, the ICH E6 Guidelines for Good Clinical Practice (GCP). ICH E6 Guidelines for GCP are legally enforceable to encourage the implementation of improved approaches to conduct clinical trial designs, data recording, and reporting. Guidelines for GCP are defined as "an international ethical and scientific quality standard for *designing*, conducting, recording, and reporting trials that involve the participation of human subjects. Compliance with this standard provides public assurance that the rights, safety and well-being of trial subjects are protected, consistent with the principles that have their origin in the Declaration of Helsinki, and that the clinical trial *data are credible*" [43] (*cursive* are mine).

In the new digital health era, in order to pursue the best treatment for a patient and make effective a medicine based on the evidence, data must be reliable and credible, and the GCP ALCOA mantra, now ALCOA ++ [44], becomes a moral imperative in order to guarantee the integrity of data: Data should be attributable, legible, contemporaneous, original, and accurate, plus complete, consistent, enduring, and available when needed, and traceable throughout the data life cycle after its creation; data are generated during their processing and are maintained or destroyed to develop new or to update drugs for emerging diseases and provide the best treatment available to the patient. The GCP skeleton consists of 13 principles with a main goal: to protect the rights and safety of patients and data reliability; therefore, the abovementioned good of the patient depends not only on the nature of each patient, but also on the data collected and processed throughout the practice of medicine across multiple patients.

Multiple scenarios showed the importance of data and big data in medicine such as artificial intelligence and its subset, machine learning. The potential benefits of big data on clinical settings are evident, resulting in preventive and personalized medicine; providing accurate diagnosis and novel therapeutic benefits; supporting development of new drugs; bringing more effective drugs to the patients; and improving vaccination effectiveness (For example, see [45, 46]). Artificial intelligence using algorithms may act in the physical or digital environment through data collected and processed to perform tasks like making decisions, may decide what is the best action, and may make predictions as well. Machine learning enabled in medical devices can create algorithms and take decisions without programming data, with an impact on the diagnosis procedure across diseases and propose treatments in patient benefit. Another novel digital technology is the new language prediction Generative Pre-trained Transformer, the so-called GPT, supporting healthcare by detecting health conditions and common symptoms, such as language impairment in patient speech using speech markers, supporting early diagnoses of neurodegenerative diseases, like dementia, among others. The use of Real Word Data is another example of the importance of data: data routinely collected from multiple sources like electronic medical records and medical devices, among others. Digital health technologies are increasing on a daily basis to guarantee the best treatment for patients in the real-world clinical settings and may support regulatory decision making and generate new guidelines for clinical practice [47].

The importance of integrity of data is also a key element in pandemic times. The coronavirus disease (COVID-19), declared as pandemic on March 11, 2020, with an enormous impact on the entire globe, especially on healthcare and clinical research, increasing demands on nurses, physicians, restrictions of study visits to the hospitals, and difficulties in distributing the drugs and investigational medicinal products, among others was a challenge for the current procedures in healthcare and clinical trials. In order to minimize the impact of COVID-19, new and updated guidelines and procedures were generated by multiple regulatory agencies like the European Medicine Agency and the Food and Drug Administration, among others, in order to facilitate decisions in benefit of patients and protect data integrity in the field of clinical research (For example, see [48–50]). The maintenance of data integrity was a key element to decide whether a clinical trial should continue despite the pandemic scenario and its difficulties or should be put on hold due to the difficulties to maintain data reliability and robustness. When it is not possible to guarantee data and their robustness, results are questioned as data are not credible, with an impact on drug development. Hence, there is no doubt data has become a *sine qua non* as digital health technologies cannot exist without data and metadata.

Indeed, the digital novel technology brings benefits in medicine, but it also may be a disruptive technology with a potential harmful impact, for example, in mental integrity or psychological profiling, by classifying groups based on their behavior and preferences, replacing human decision-making, among others [51], and also potential misuses via security, economic or politics. Ransomware attacks on hospitals for business purposes have increased, with a direct impact on healthcare [52], algorithms may predict criminal recidivism [53] and may involve risks of stigmatization or discrimination in societies, or spyware tools designed to secretly turn mobile phones phones into means of repression means of repression, with an impact on the privacy of Presidents, legislators, and members of civil society organizations, as occurred in the Pegasus case (e.g., see the Pegasus case [54]), putting in question the protection of the confidentiality and privacy of political opinions, philosophical beliefs, and personal data, although protected by multiple regulations [55, 56].

Digital health technologies bring benefits and risks, thanks to their systems and algorithms creating multiple complex scenarios based on data gathered, and their metadata, during the entire data life cycle. However, as principles have an inherent limitation, data also have their inherent limitation: Algorithms are learning on the basis of historical data entered in multiple sources by humans with their values and preferences and access to computers; therefore, data gathered contain biases and mistakes. However, despite the inherent limitation, data are used and processed. Data are not virtual and are real, and as the mantra says: If something is not documented, it does not exist; if facts are not documented, it did not happen; in other words, data are moral content *per se*.

4. Conclusion: bioethics by-design

As stated by Edmund Pincoffs, the nature of time dictates what ethics there must be [3]. Indeed, bioethics is linked to the current times, and this is not an exception in the current digital era. In medicine, despite the advantages of novel digital technologies, the impact on patients and society is still unknown. Digital technologies and the added moral content, data, raise novel ethical challenges and bring new ethics debates at all stages of the data life cycle, from their creation, use, and management, until they are destroyed. Data are registered in millions of systems through multiple sources such as internet browsers, applications, online platforms, and devices, among others, and then are processed, analyzed, and controlled through multiple systems and procedures until they are destroyed or saved for future process, increasing zettabytes of data with their biases.

In April 2019, the EU's High-Level Expert Group (HLEG) on artificial intelligence published its Ethical Guidelines, identifying key requirements that artificial intelligence systems should meet to be trustworthy. Among them, human oversight, data governance, and principles of bioethics like the principle of autonomy or the principle of nonmaleficence have been adopted as ethical guideline [57]. Indeed, bioethical principles help create a common discourse between by facilitating a *lingua franca* and an interdisciplinary dialog as stated by E. Pellegrino [22]; however, data and their algorithms require human oversight and data governance to avoid their potential misuse in medicine, sociology, politics, and across human disciplines in general.

At present, changes in healthcare management and organization, the creation of new hospital complexes, changes in morbidity, the increase in chronic diseases, greater longevity, the increase in home care and decentralized clinical trials, the existence of patients with multiple pathologies that require the intervention of different teams and different specialties, plus the impact of digital technologies on health, are generating ethical conflicts that have more to do with organization, resource management, systems, and data than with clinical practice itself. Thus, ethics consultants and ethics committees must deal with issues that are related to the structure and functioning of healthcare organizations; the well-functioning of digital technologies, however, may not yet be ready to address the new emerging ethical conflicts raised or having the root cause in systems and algorithms.

While the era when ethics consultation was immersed into organizational ethics was defined as the second stage of bioethics [58, 59], the current digital era brings the bioethics community to a third stage. While during the second stage, issues occurring in medicine had an organizational nature and were closely linked to the management of resources, now issues are systems and design related, linked to the nature of data.

Since the implementation of ethics committees in hospitals, the debate on which profile is the most suitable to be part of it has been a constant. It was a dispute whether philosophers or physicians are recommended to deal with ethical issues in the practice of medicine. The majority of surveys showed that physicians and nurses were the groups with the most representatives on ethics committees in the US, in detriment of other profiles such as social workers, psychologists, lawyers, or philosophers [60–63]. In the digital era, the role of the Data Privacy Office has been established in multiple organizations as a result of the implementation of multiple regulations, and the same question can be raised: Who is the most preferable profile to guarantee data are processed and controlled as expected during their entire life cycle? Knowledge on data protection law seems to be a prerequisite, plus communication skills, and preferably knowledge of information technologies, including security and organizational aspects [64], but given the increase of novel digital technologies and their potential misuse, we are forced to continue investigating about the best skills, knowledge, and abilities needed to properly address novel issues in the digital era.

In the second stage of bioethics, given the need to deal with aspects of an organizational nature, ethics consultants and committees were forced to rethink their approach. If at the first stage of bioethics, the main task of the ethic consultants and ethics committees was directed to the resolution of ethical issues, with a reactive attitude, the second stage has been marked by the ethics of the organizations, with a more preventive attitude, and the function of the committees was more focused to the prevention of ethical issues, rather than its resolution; this was possible by efforts made toward training and promoting an ethics that encompasses clinical ethics and the ethics of the organization. The jump from clinical ethics to organizational ethics not only entailed changes in the structure of ethics committees, but also impacted their functions. In the current digital era, multiple procedures and systems have been established, and trainings seem not to be sufficient either to solve or to prevent issues due to the complexity and recurrence of novel issues. In the digital era, issues are not always related to the human nature, nor to the organization nature, but in the system and its design. Thus, the third bioethics stage cannot be limited to a reactive approach or preventive approach, but efforts must be made to adopt a proactive approach to avoid errors in systems or process where data gathered are managed and used by algorithms to make decisions with a direct or indirect impact on humans, in medicine, patients.

In other words, bioethics and their main tool, ethics consultants, and ethics committees, changed upon the context within which it operates, and required knowledge, skills, and abilities are changing as well. As stated by the UNESCO, because we are living in digitalizing society, responsible design practices and new skills are required [46, 65]. If in the second stage of bioethics, knowledge about organization structure or business by ethics consultants was questioned; in this third stage, without minimal knowledge and skills of digital technologies, ethics consultants and also regulators may have difficulties to manage the new emerging issues properly and propose adequate ethical guidelines and regulations. In medicine, a third element has been incorporated to the nature of the patient and the nature of the organizations: the nature of systems. The good and right decision depends on the human nature, on the compliance to procedures, and the good design of systems governing data gathered and created by humans and non-humans. Thus, in clinical bioethics, the moral responsibility to make good decisions not only falls on healthcare professionals or procedure, but also falls on the system and its design, to guarantee outcomes to benefit the patient. A new third approach is required, which may be called integrative bioethics by-design.

Integrative, both procedural and substantive approaches, bioethics should be the centric approach to how systems should be designed without omitting the real and cyber moral content and its context. As stated by experts, artificial intelligence can be trustworthy if the system, during its entire life cycle, is "ethical, ensuring adherence to ethical principles and values" [57], and systems should be designed in order to be able to respect and implement bioethics and data protection principles by-design, and by default to meet requirements of current regulations and ethical guidelines. If the essential trait of the procedural bioethics approach is that it focuses on the formulation of procedures that help solve issues while respecting principles, the essential trait of integrative bioethics by-design approach is it focuses on the generation of systems to allow procedures to solve issues in the current digital era while respecting bioethics and data privacy principles. The impact of novel digital technologies applied in health is still unknown, and an integrative bioethics by-design approach may support bioethicists and experts on systems and digital technology to make the right and good decision; meanwhile, regulations and guidelines need to be developed and put into effect across human disciplines, like medicine, and multiple fields.

Patients, organizations, and systems are interrelated and complement each other being difficult to work separately. While the substantive bioethics approach provides content, and principlism and the procedural approach provide normativity, integrative bioethics by-design provides ethical robustness to the systems. Errors are inherent to humans, gaps are inherent to the procedures, and both process gaps and human errors are inherent to the systems and as such can be avoided by an integrative bioethics by-design approach by providing the right approach to systems throughout their development. Systems, like procedures, have their inherent ingenuity, and an integrative bioethics by-design approach may overcome system ingenuity, as substantive bioethics approach overcomes the procedural ingenuity. While the substantive approach provides content, and the procedural approach provides normativity, integrative bioethics by-design provides normativity while respecting substantive approach.

When developing regulations for digital technologies and systems, integrative bioethics by-design must be considered as technological readiness level is considered when new technologies are developed prior to their implementation. The integrative bioethics by-design approach may guarantee bioethics principles are respected and linked properly to the systems and algorithms during the entire life cycle, having an impact on their correct use.

After what has been said, we can conclude that procedural, substantive, and integrative by-design approaches are and must be interrelated to deal with the new emerging ethical dilemmas in the digital era. From now on, a new mantra is coming: bioethics by-design.

Notes

The beginning of our research started from a personal interest in the physician-patient relationship. After a bibliographical review on the subject and reading texts on medical history, ethics, and anthropology, we realized that concepts such as "trust," "virtue," or the "good of the patient" are essential as the basis for an ethics of medicine. This is where our interest in virtue ethics and Aristotle's ethical theory came from, given its constant allusion to the practice of medicine and because is one of the most important references in the debate on the concept of "virtue." At that point, there were two decisive factors that influenced the direction of our research:

the observation of the defenders of virtue ethics that for a long period of time, the concept of virtue in contemporary ethical theories became a forgotten concept, giving greater importance to other concepts of ethics such as "duty" or the "consequences," and the formulation of and impact on the development of the bioethical discourse of the four bioethics principles of Tom L. Beauchamp and James F. Childress. We therefore wanted to delve deeper into different bioethical theories, such as that of Robert M. Veatch and Hugo T. Engelhardt and in the philosophy of medicine by Edmund D. Pellegrino and David C. Thomasma, to determine whether or not the impact of proceduralism on bioethics led to a forgetfulness of content or virtue.

The digital era brings benefits and risks thanks to their systems and algorithms, creating multiple complex scenarios and requiring a third key approach: by-design.

Author details

Salvador Ribas Ribas
Independent Ethics Advisor, Doctor of Philosophy, Barcelona, Spain

*Address all correspondence to: salvador.ribas@gmail.com

References

[1] Callahan D. Bioethics as a discipline. Hastings Center Studies. 1973;**1**(1):66-73

[2] Kass N, Dawson L, Loyo-Berrios NI. Ethical oversight of research in developing countries. IRB Ethics & Human Research. 2003;**25**(2):1-10

[3] Pincoffs EL. Quandary ethics. Mind. 1971;**80**(320):552-571

[4] Siegler M. The progression of medicine. From physician paternalism to patient autonomy to bureaucratic parsimony. Archives of Internal Medicine. 1985;**145**:713-715

[5] Alexander S. They decide who lives, who dies. Life. 1962;**9**:103-125

[6] The National Commission for the Protection of Human Subjects of Biomedical and Behavioral Research. The Belmont Report: Ethical Principles and Guidelines for the Protection of Human Subjects of Research. Washington DC: Department of Health, Education, and Welfare; 1979

[7] Beauchamp TL, Childress JF. Principles of Biomedical Ethics. New York: Oxford University Press; 1979

[8] Veatch RM. A Theory of Medical Ethics. New York: Basic Books; 1981

[9] Engelhardt TH. The Foundations of Bioethics. New York: Oxford University Press; 1986

[10] Veatch RM. Professional medical ethics: The grounding of its principles. Journal of Medicine and Philosophy. 1979;**4**(1):1-19

[11] Becker L. The neglect of virtue. Ethics. 1975;**85**(2):110-122

[12] Anscombe GEM. Modern moral philosophy. Philosophy. 1958;**33**(124):1-19

[13] Hursthouse R. On virtue ethics. Oxford: Oxford University Press; 1999. p. 25

[14] Drane JF. Becoming a Good Doctors. The Place of Virtue in Medical Ethics. Kansas City: Sheed and Ward; 1995

[15] Pellegrino ED, Thomasma DC. The Virtues in Medical Practice. New York: Oxford University Press; 1993

[16] Pellegrino ED. Medical ethics: Entering the post-hippocratic era. Journal of the American Board of Family Practice. 1988;**1**(4):230-237

[17] Jonsen AR, Siegler M, Winslade WJ. Clinical Ethics. A Practical Approach to Ethical Decisions in Clinical Medicine. 2nd ed. New York: Macmillan Publishing Company; 1986

[18] Tong R. Feminist Approaches to Bioethics: Theoretical Reflections and Practical Applications. Boulder: Westview Press; 1997

[19] McGee G, editor. Pragmatic Bioethics. Nashville: Vanderbilt University Press; 1999

[20] Frankena WK. Ethics. Englewood Cliffs: Prentice-Hall; 1973. p. 65

[21] Beauchamp TL. Principlism and its alleged competitors. Kennedy Institute of Ethics Journal. 1995;**5**(3):181-198

[22] Pellegrino ED. The four principles and the doctor-patient relationship: The need for a better linkage. In: Gillon R, editor. Principles of Health Care Ethics.

New York: John Wiley and Sons; 1994. p. 360

[23] Kass LR. Practicing ethics: where's the action. Hastings Center Report. 1990;**20**(1):5-12

[24] Brody H. The physician-patient relationships: models and criticism. Theoretical Medicine and Bioethics. 1987;**8**(2):205-220

[25] Childress JF. Who should decide? Paternalism in health care. New York: Oxford University Press; 1982. p. 6

[26] Childress JF, Siegler M. Metaphors and models of doctor-patient relationships: their implications for autonomy. Theoretical Medicine and Bioethics. 1984;**5**(1):16-30

[27] Emanuel EJ, Emanuel LL. Four models of the physician-patient relationship. Journal of the American Medical Association. 1992;**267**(16):2221-2226

[28] Thomasma DC. Beyond medical paternalism and patient autonomy: a model of physician conscience for the physician-patient relationship. Annals of Internal Medicine. 1983;**98**(2):243-248

[29] Thomasma DC. Models of the doctor-patient relationship and the ethics committee: part one. Cambridge Quarterly of Healthcare Ethics. 1992;**1**(1):11-31

[30] Thomasma DC. Models of the doctor-patient relationship and the ethics committee: part two. Cambridge Quarterly of Healthcare Ethics. 1994;**3**(1):10-26

[31] Ozar DT. Patients' autonomy: three models of the professional-lay relationship in medicine. Theoretical Medicine and Bioethics. 1984;**5**(1):61-68

[32] Veatch RM. Models for ethical medicine in a revolutionary age. Hastings Center Report. 1972;**2**(3):5-7

[33] Brennan TA. Ethics committees and decisions to limit care. The experience at the Massachusetts General Hospital. Journal of the American Medical Association. 1988;**260**(6):803-807

[34] Supreme Court of New Jersey. In re Quinlan. In the matter of Karen Quinlan. 1976.355 A.2d.647 (N.J.)

[35] US Government Printing Office. President's Commission for the Study of Ethical Problems in Medicine and Biomedical and Behavioral Research. Deciding to Forego Life Sustaining Treatment. Washington DC: US Government Printing Office; 1983. pp. 160-170

[36] American Hospital Association. Guidelines. Hospital Committees on Biomedical Ethics. Chicago: American Hospital Association; 1984

[37] American Medical Association. Judicial council. Guidelines for ethics committees in health care institutions. Journal of the American Medical Association. 1985;**253**(18):2698-2699

[38] Carter BS. A survey of army clinicians on hospital ethics committees. Military Medicine. 1989;**154**(8):392-394

[39] Finkenbine R, Gramelspacher G. Physicians' attitudes toward hospitals ethics committees. Indiana Medicine. 1991;**84**:804-807

[40] Youngner SJ, Coulton C, Juknilais BW, Jackson DL. Patients' attitudes toward hospital ethics committees. Law, Medicine and Health Care. 1984;**12**(1):21-25

[41] Ribas S. Las competencias de los Comités de Ética Asistencial y la autoevaluación de sus componentes.

El estudio CEA-CAT (2). Medicina Clínica. 2007;**6**(186):219-225. DOI: 10.1157/13098718

[42] This was already stated by The Economist. 2017. Available from: https://www.economist.com. [Accessed April 26, 2023]

[43] ICH Guideline E6(R2) Guideline for Good Clinical Practice. The ICH E6 (R1) GCP was published in 1996, and it was amended in 2016 with guideline E6 (R2) being effective in June 2017. Currentl, E6 R3 is under review. 2016

[44] EMA. Good Clinical Practice Inspectors Working Group. Guideline on computerised systems and electronic data in clinical trials. EMA/INS/GCP/112288/2023, p. 13; 2023

[45] Pelčić G, Ribas S, Coha A, Tucak I, Vuletić S, Pavlinović S, Valković A: The place of big data in addressing emerged issues in vaccinology of the 21st century. JAHR European Journal of Bioethics 2020;11(2):335-355 10.21860/j.11.2.1

[46] FDA. Using artificial intelligence and machine learning in the development of drug and biological product. Discussion paper and request for feedback. 2023. Available from: https://www.fda.gov/media/167973/download. [Accessed May 11, 2023]

[47] For information about the impact of Real World Data in the medicine see https://www.fda.gov/science-research/science-and-research-special-topics/real-world-evidence. [Accessed April 26, 2023]

[48] EMA. Guidance on the Management of Clinical Trials during the COVID 19 (Coronavirus) pandemic, version 1.0, March 20, 2020; version 2.0, March 27, 2020; and version 3.0, April 28, 2020. 2020

[49] European Data Protection Board. Guidelines 03/2020 on the processing of data concerning health for the purpose of scientific research in the context of the COVID-19 outbreak. 2020. Adopted April 21, 2020

[50] FDA Guidance on Conduct of Clinical Trials of Medical Products during COVID-19 Pandemic. Guidance for Industry, Investigators, and Institutional Review Boards, March 2020, and updated on March 27, April 2, April 16, May 11, May 14, June 3, and July 2, 2020. 2020

[51] Federspiel F, Mitchell R, Asokan A, Umana C, McCoy D. Threats by artificial intelligence to human health and human existence. BMJ Global Health. 2023;**8**:010435. DOI: 10.1136/bmjgh-2022-010435

[52] Neprash HT, McGlave CC, Cross DA, Virnig BA, Puskarich MA, Huling JD, Rozenshtein AZ, Nikpay SS: Trends in ransomware attacks on US hospitals, clinics, and other health care delivery organizations, 2016-2021. JAMA Health Forum. 2022; 3(12): e224873. 10.1001/jamahealthforum.2022.4873. Available from: https://jamanetwork.com/journals/jama-health-forum/fullarticle/2799961. [Accessed May 9, 2023]

[53] Tolan S, Miron M, Gomez E, Castillo C. Why machine learning may Lead to unfairness: Evidence from risk assessment for juvenile justice in Catalonia. Best Paper Award, Proceedings of the Seventeenth International Conference on Artificial Intelligence and Law. 2019;**2019**:83-92. DOI: 10.1145/3322640.3326705

[54] Marzocchi O. Pegasus and surveillance spyware Pegasus case. European Parliament. 2022

[55] Regulation (EU) 2016/679 of the European Parliament and of the Council

of 27 April 2016 on the protection of natural persons with regard to the processing of personal data and on the free movement of such data

[56] Council of Europe Convention 108+. Convention for the protection of individuals with regard to the processing of personal data. Council of Europe. 2018

[57] European Commission. Independent High-Level Expert Group on Artificial Intelligence. Ethics guidelines for trustworthy AI. Brussels. 2019. Available from: https://ec.europa.eu/digital-single-market/en/high-level-expert-group-artificial-intelligence. [Accessed May 9, 2023]

[58] Potter RL. From clinical ethics to organizational ethics: The second stage of the evolution of bioethics. Bioethics Forum. 1996;**1996**:3-12

[59] Simón P. La ética de las organizaciones sanitarias: el segundo estadio de desarrollo de la bioética. Revista de Calidad Asistencial. 2002;**17**(4):247-259

[60] Marsh FH. Why physicians should not do ethics consults. Theoretical Medicine and Bioethics. 1992;**13**(3):285-292

[61] Ruddick W. Can doctors and philosophers work together? Hastings Center Report. 1981;**11**(2):12-17

[62] Ruddick W, Finn W. Objections to hospital philosophers. Journal of Medical Ethics. 1985;**11**(1):42-46

[63] Ribas S. Healthcare Ethics Committees in US: Bibliographic Review. Barcelona: Institut Borja de Bioética-Fundación Mapfre Medicina; 2003

[64] European Data Protection Supervisor. Position Paper on the Role of Data Protection Officers in Ensuring Effective Compliance with Regulation (EC) 45/2001. Brussels: European Data Protection Supervisor; 2005

[65] UNESCO. Recommendation on the Ethics of Artificial Intelligence. Paris: UNESCO; 2022

Chapter 11

Bioethics in Laboratory Medicine

Ashish P. Anjankar, Namrata Anjankar and Vaibhav Anjankar

Abstract

Medical laboratory professionals are answerable to the ethical codes of their profession. This idea also holds for laboratory medicine. All patients should be treated equally and without distinction in the laboratory. Data gathering for the accurate patient and specimen identification is where laboratory medicine ethics begin. Ethical principles are upheld when gathering samples, conducting the tests, and disclosing the results. When a patient presents themselves at a lab with a request form and readily consents to the standard collecting procedures, consent can be assumed for most laboratory procedures. The laboratory must always conduct tests by the relevant standards. Laboratory test results are kept private unless disclosure is permitted. The results will typically be reported to the requesting doctor, with the patient's permission or as required by law; they may also be reported to other parties. Medical records should be stored and kept following ethical standards. Instead of being spelled out in an operating manual, laboratory staff members must uphold ethics in laboratory medicine. This calls for medical laboratory professionals to be aware of their responsibilities and diligently approach their work.

Keywords: bioethics, laboratory medicine, laboratory physicians, patient care, ethical standards

1. Introduction

A set of moral guidelines, medical ethics, applies ethical standards to clinical medicine and scientific research. Professionals can turn to a group of values that form the foundation of medical ethics in case of any uncertainty or conflict. These values include respect for one's autonomy, beneficence, justice, trustworthiness, and non-maleficence.

2. Bioethics in laboratory medicine

The duty of medical doctors to their patients is to follow their professional skills ethically and to observe the laws of the community. The purpose is to justify the patient's trust in the medical profession. Like other areas of medicine, laboratory medicine is also committed to high ethical standards. The patient's welfare is paramount in healthcare ethics. This principle applies to laboratory medicine as well.

Medical laboratory professionals are answerable to the ethical codes of their profession. The general principle of healthcare ethics is that the patient's welfare is paramount. The laboratory should treat all patients fairly and without discrimination.

The three main groups medical laboratories are responsible for our patients, coworkers, and society. The expected behavior of laboratory physicians is defined as "ethical medical practice," and striving to uphold the highest ethical standards is crucial for advancing medicine [1]. Maintaining their professional integrity is laboratory doctors' main priority.

3. Why is ethics important in laboratory medicine?

Currently, lab testing makes up about 70% of medical diagnoses [2]. This accentuates the crucial role that laboratory physicians play in patient care. The intermediary clinician, acting as the patient's lawyer, must endorse the same ethical framework as the laboratory physician to ensure that investigation results are practiced in the patient's best interest. Verdicts about diagnosis, prognosis, and treatment are frequently based on the results and interpretations of laboratory tests [3, 4].

Clinical laboratories must consider ethical considerations when gathering patient data, collecting samples, performing tests, stocking samples, following storage protocol, and keeping records. Other ethical issues surrounding clinical laboratories include those unrelated to patients such as managing biomedical waste and financial arrangements.

Several countries and professional organizations have developed guidelines on ethical issues related to laboratory medicine. For instance, the International Organization for Standardization (ISO) has created ISO 15189:2012, "Medical laboratories — Requirements for quality and competence" [5]. Many professional societies have defined codes of ethics for laboratory professionals [6–11].

Although the importance of ethics in laboratory medicine is undisputed, there is volatility in education that is concentrated on ethics in laboratory medicine. The IFCC task force has recommended that all medical specialties, including laboratory medicine, should adhere to ethical standards and guidelines. The outcome, results, and analysis of laboratory tests are typically used to determine prognosis and medications associated with specific medical conditions.

Laboratory professionals face ethical dilemmas daily, but ethics needs to receive the attention it deserves. A report by the International Federation of Clinical Chemistry and Laboratory Medicine Task Force on Ethics shows that many laboratory medicine training programs do not formally teach ethics and that there is a need for training programs for ethical considerations in laboratory medicine.

Clinical laboratories must consider ethical considerations when gathering patient information, collecting specimens, performing tests, stocking samples, following storage protocol for results reporting, and keeping records. There are several other areas of ethical concern related to clinical laboratories such as biomedical waste management and financial arrangements, which are not directly related to patients [12].

3.1 Basic ethical principles in the pre-analytical phase

3.1.1 Collection of information

Ethics in laboratory medicine commence from collecting information for proper recognition of patients and specimens. The laboratory should collect sufficient information to correctly identify the patient and representative. The Clinical and Laboratory Standard Institute (CLSI) makes suggestions for enhancing the precision of inpatient and outpatient identification. In accordance with CLSI guidelines, inpatients should be asked for their complete name, address, birthdate, age, and/or unique identification number.

Although it is also legal (for billing and the security of other patients), irrelevant personal information should not be gathered. The patient should be informed of the reason behind the data collection [13, 14].

3.1.2 Collection of specimen

Consent can be assumed for most laboratory procedures when patients present themselves at the lab with a request form and readily consents to standard data collection techniques such as venipuncture. Unique methods, such as those that are more invasive (such as bone marrow aspirations), call for a more thorough explanation and, occasionally, written consent. Adequate privacy for the patient must be made available (type of specimen collected).

Sample collection should be carried out following generally accepted safety precautions to protect both the patient and the healthcare professional. Additional samples should not be taken from patients without informing the institution's ethics committee and receiving their permission. The specimens need to be clearly labeled. The integrity of the sample should be protected during transportation.

Specimen integrity is the second most important prerequisite for lowering laboratory error during the pre-analytical phase. The amount of procedures carried out, such as specimen collecting, specimen physiology maintenance, transportation, and processing, affect the integrity of the specimen. The actions listed below will guarantee specimen integrity:

The laboratory should develop simple-to-understand procedures for gathering, handling, and transporting samples. Standard operating protocols (SOPs) for phlebotomy must be followed by the laboratory, and they cover things like the right way to collect samples, how to take the necessary safety precautions when collecting samples, and how to dispose of syringes, needles, and other supplies.

The only way to do this is to go through training, which starts at the new employee orientation period and includes a continuing education program that is completed annually or as needed, followed by an annual proficiency and competency exam. All non-laboratory and laboratory staff involved in specimen collecting should receive this training.

To ensure the validity of analytical results, laboratories should establish evidence-based standards for specimen acceptance that must be put into practice for managing the specimens prior to testing [11]. A standardized workflow for identifying and handling hemolyzed, clotted, and inadequate specimen material should be developed by laboratories.

Counseling will be required for human immunodeficiency virus (H.I.V.) testing and specific genetic testing such as hereditary cancer genetic test, prenatal genetic test, and genome screening. In emergencies, consent is not possible, and under these circumstances, it is sufficient to perform necessary procedures, provided they are in the patient's best interest. Laboratories performing H.I.V. testing shall pursue the National AIDS Control Organization guidelines, which include pretest and posttest counseling. Specific genetic testing will require pretest counseling to ensure the patient fully realizes the significance of the test result [15–17].

3.1.3 Patient autonomy

The patient's right to refuse to be tested should be respected. However, in certain situations, the patient's autonomy is not absolute. For instance, when the patient is unconscious, mentally ill, or under the influence of drugs, they may be presumed incapable of deciding their health. Schedule-Y, FDA, ICH-GCP, WHO, and ICMR guidelines all list vulnerable populations as including low-income individuals, patients who are illiterate, children, patients in psychiatric facilities, inmates, fetuses, and pregnant women. Children are generally not supposed to make decisions for them. When a patient is incompetent for a reason (age or mental state), consent may be given by a parent or other authorized proxy.

Poor women with HIV/AIDS are one such susceptible group; on occasion, these participants are not aware of the process of informed consent. Many researchers lament that because respondents have varied perceptions of diseases, it might be challenging to explain the study's biological foundation and treatment plans to them. However, this should not be the justification for not getting subjects' informed consent. In order to better comprehend the informed consent process and HIV/AIDS, developing nations such as India conduct Group Education and Counseling (GEC). Through seminars and questionnaires, fundamental information on HIV/AIDS and the informed consent process was imparted. Many individuals could comprehend the significance of informed consent with only a small amount of education, and occasionally it is important to abandon the traditional paradigm in favor of a new one.

Specific populations, including intravenous drug users and prisoners, require mandatory testing. In these exceptional circumstances, laboratory professionals have a responsibility to consider the policies set forth by the organization in which they work and to balance the advantages of the testing against the risks of a patient's autonomy is lost.

It offers affordable access to several laboratory tests. When better tests are available, the laboratory should assess whether it is necessary to discontinue older tests and whether any opportunities exist to replace them. No patients should be given preference to simplify or speed up the collection process at the expense of other patients.

3.2 Analytical phase

3.2.1 Performance of tests

The laboratory shall always use test procedures, which meet the applicable standards. The preferred methods have been documented in reputable, peer reviewed textbooks, texts, or journals and in international, national, or regional guidelines. If internal processes are used, they must be thoroughly documented and validated adequately for their intended use.

The laboratory is accountable for meticulously reporting laboratory results and ensuring that the results are correctly interpreted and used in the patient's best interests. In some situations, the laboratory should refuse to attempt a test rather than produce an unreliable result that could harm the patient. The maxim "a wrong result is worse than no result" is a guiding principle.

Good laboratory practice includes the refusal to analyze or report a result when evidence of deficiencies may compromise the test result. All laboratory work must be carried out with a high level of skill and competence expected of the medical, scientific, and allied health professions.

Patients can decline to have their samples examined after sample collection and processing. Confidentiality should be respected and maintained in such a situation. To the greatest extent possible, confidentiality should be respected during point-of-care testing.

3.3 Post-analytical phase

This phase includes reporting and interpreting test results, storing residual samples, and accessing the data.

3.3.1 Reporting of results

The requesting clinician will typically receive a report of the findings. The patient's permission, or as required by law, may be obtained to disclose the results to other parties. The laboratory should have written policies outlining how different requests are to be handled, and patients should have access to this information upon request.

Although reporting of test results must be consistent for all patients, speedy reporting may be demanded some results including "critical" and "significant risk" results. The International Federation of Biomedical Laboratory Science (I.F.B.L.S.) suggests upholding strict confidentiality of patient data and test results, protecting patients' privacy and dignity, and, most importantly, taking responsibility for the caliber and integrity of clinical laboratory services rendered. Similarly, the American Society of Clinical Pathologists (A.S.C.P.) has also given laboratory staff advice on how to treat patients and coworkers with respect, care, and consideration; how to perform tasks accurately, precisely, promptly, and responsibly; and how to keep patient information private while adhering to the law. Laboratory test results are kept confidential unless disclosure is permitted by law, under exceptional circumstances, or both. For instance [18, 19]:

1. When sending a patient to another hospital.

2. When a court or the police issue a written request requesting.

3. By the Insurance Act, the insurance provider must obtain the patient's reports when the patient waives their right to get insurance.

4. When required by consumer protection and workers' compensation laws.

5. Notification of disease through disease registration.

6. Research into infectious diseases.

7. Studies on vaccination.

8. Reporting of adverse drug reactions.

9. By the Right to Information Act, a person's medical records should be made public if admitted to a government hospital while in police or judicial custody.

The laboratory is also responsible for taking all necessary precautions to guarantee the security and dependability of the method of transmitting results to interested clinicians and other authorized parties. A quality reporting system is one that makes sure the right results are sent to the right medical practitioners in a timely manner that assures patient safety without placing an undue strain on the medical staff or the laboratory staff [20]. According to the definition of this system, two crucial flaws could endanger patient safety if they are not resolved. First is "delivering the report within a time frame" and second is "delivery to the appropriate [health care professional]." Regarding the first concern, the reporting of critical values—defined as values that represent circumstances that could become life-threatening unless some kind of medical intervention is made and for which such interventions are feasible—may offer a particularly significant risk to patient safety. It is also important to consider the second issue, "delivery to the appropriate [health care professional]," which has to do with who should be informed and who should receive test results.

Whether the transmission occurs *via* electronic, postal, or courier service, decisions concerning implied consent for reporting results to other practitioners involved (such as consultant practitioners to whom the patient has been referred) should be made carefully, considering local customs.

The laboratory is also liable for ensuring that the turnaround time for results is acceptable, considering the type of test and the patient's condition. Urgent results should be reported as soon as they are available. The facility should be to report critical results as soon as they are available. Reporting delays ought to be prevented. Inaccurate outcomes can result in poor management. Errors should be reported to ordering clinicians as soon as they are discovered, and test results should be updated as quickly as possible. The modification on the report should be noted, and any incorrect results should be clearly labeled. The laboratory has to ensure that the results are correctly interpreted and used in the patient's best interest, in addition, to accurately reporting the results of the tests.

A competent professional's consultation regarding the selection and interpretation of the results is a part of medical laboratory service. The results of laboratory examinations that have been detached from all patient identification may be used for purposes such as epidemiology, demography, or other statistical analyses.

Because the patient has not paid, withholding laboratory results should be avoided. A policy on the use of residual samples should be developed. Residual models are often used without the patient's knowledge. There is a dilemma about patients' profit share if financial gains are derived from leftover samples. Fleischman argues that the most crucial concern surrounding remaining dried blood spots now is whether they may be preserved and utilized for upcoming studies without endangering the crucial public health objectives of newborn screening programs. Yes, he replied, "as long as we exercise caution."

Would it be a breach of confidentially if we discovered the patient had a certain genetic condition for which he or she had not given consent to a genetic test and this was actionable? "Genetic exceptionalism" refers to the notion that genetic testing is distinct from testing for other illnesses [18]. Genetic data is personal and directly relates to a person's identity. The results of a genetic test may have an impact on the entire family, making confidentiality a problem not only for work but also for medical care. If a person has or is genetically predisposed to the condition, that person's parents, children, siblings, and even extended relatives may also be afflicted. A person may also rely important decisions on the results of a genetic test [21].

3.3.2 Storage and retention of medical records

All of the records should be organized, easily readable, and stored in a convenient location. Test results must only be changed or corrected if done so by legally qualified individuals following established protocols. Facilities must create a suitable environment to guard against loss, devaluation, destruction, and unauthorized access. According to national, regional, or local legal regulations, records may be kept for a convenient retention period. Laboratories should develop protocols indicating retention time for different results, specimens, and slides. Test results should be physically available for ready authorized access. When medical records must be destroyed, this should be carried out with the minimal risk of inadvertent disclosure. The following techniques can be used to destroy paper records: burning, shredding, pulping, and pulverizing. Destruction techniques for microfilm or microfiche include recycling and pulverizing.

3.3.3 Access to medical records

Access should be available to the clinicians, patients, hospital staff, and other authorized individuals. The laboratory should develop protocols to handle special requests considering local laws and customs. The person's identity must be confirmed by the laboratory when an authorized person requests to access the result. In exceptional circumstances, the prohibition of health information from individuals usually authorized to receive it may be justified. An example of such a circumstance is when disclosure may be contrary to a patient's best interests.

For various tests, different techniques might be used in the same laboratory. For instance, an authorized person requesting the results of an H.I.V. test may be required to provide much more proof of their identity than someone asking for the results of a routine hemoglobin test. For each circumstance, laboratories should establish the proper protocols.

3.3.4 Financial arrangements

When financial agreements with referring clinicians motivate patient referrals, medical laboratories should not enter into those agreements. Private laboratory collection rooms should be entirely independent of the rooms used by the referring clinicians. Any financial arrangements must only include an element of encouragement if this is feasible. Laboratories must be able to function independently and try to avoid situations that could lead to conflicts of interest.

3.3.5 Conscientiousness of the laboratory personnel

- The laboratory personnel must assess his/her conduct and maintain professional integrity.

- The personnel must take great care in performing the test procedure and recording the results.

- The patient's sample must be carefully stored.

- No fabrication (Unauthorized altering or falsification of data) of the sample to be tested or the result should be done.

- While delegating tasks to the staff, great care has to be taken, keeping in mind the importance of each patient's sample.
- Financial or personal interests should not supersede the patient's welfare.

3.3.6 Research ethics

As science and modern medicine continue to advance, new moral and ethical dilemmas frequently appear. The human genome project's completion, the expansion of genetic engineering, and stem cell research are just a few examples of things that are at the forefront of ethical discussions today. The focus on ethical misconduct in the media and the growing scrutiny of science's intricate financial ties to business and industry both serve to emphasize the importance of ethics in scientific conduct. We as scientists must develop our moral and ethical character because science ethics are becoming more and more important.

According to the researcher, the patient's informed consent must be obtained before using any samples. Without fabricating (Unauthorized altering or falsification of data) any reports, the researcher must accurately report the information, tools, and techniques used in the lab. The confidentiality of patient data gathered for research purposes must be upheld at all times by the researcher.

3.3.7 Histopathology and cytology

Specific observations (such as the presence of spermatozoa) that are unrelated to the examination's goal may be made during a histopathological or cytological assessment. It is essential to carefully consider whether or not to report such observations because doing so could have critical social repercussions.

Like clinical pathology, tissue diagnosis must offer details that help the treating physician properly inform the patient of the diagnosis and its repercussions.

3.3.8 Reproductive technology

Discussions of reproductive technology may bring up issues that touch on deeply held beliefs and religious principles, as well as perceptions of what it means to be a human being or a person, about identity, about the family, and the idea that one's traits continue to exist in some way after death.

Judaism permits the use of all assisted reproductive technologies when the oocyte and spermatozoon come from the husband and wife, respectively. Among Christian groups, there are differences in attitudes toward reproductive practices. Even though the Vatican does not support assisted reproduction, Protestant, Anglican, and other religious groups may use it. The majority of assisted reproductive technologies are prohibited by traditional Christian beliefs because they hold that the embryo has moral status as a human being from the moment of conception. IVF and embryo transfer are acceptable in Islam, but they are only permitted for husband and wife to use them. New religious questions are posed by advances in science and technology, along with the clinical applications that follow, often without clear-cut solutions.

The way various societies and religions approach these issues varies, just as do these convictions and perceptions. As a result, it is impossible to reach a consensus among ethical thinkers on this issue. Examples of this concern are the various and firmly held opinions on artificial insemination by donors, *in vitro* fertilization, gamete intrafallopian transfer, and other procedures and techniques.

3.3.9 Recommendation for ethical practices in a laboratory

- Standardization of all procedures.
- Safe environment including proper wiring and upkeep of all electrical appliances and diagnostic equipment.
- Administration assurance of the safety of the laboratory staff from healthcare risks.
- Automation including bar coding that decreases manual error.
- Different tiers of checking/monitoring systems to detect the errors promptly.
- Repeated training of the staff.
- Reducing distractions such as mobile devices.

4. Conclusion

Medical mistakes typically occur when a planned action is not carried out as intended or when the wrong plan is carried out. Instead of being spelled out in an operating manual, laboratory staff members must uphold ethics in laboratory medicine. To achieve this, medical laboratory professionals must be aware of their responsibilities and diligently approach their work. For ethical practice, the laboratory physician must never forget the fundamental virtues of compassion, discernment, trustworthiness, integrity, and conscientiousness. It is necessary to create an ethics policy for laboratory professionals (similar to code of conduct for various companies or business) and include it in the quality control manual for the laboratory. The code of ethics usually includes the six universal moral values that state you expect employees to be trustworthy, respectful, responsible, fair, caring, and good citizens. The creation and implementation of an ethics training program for laboratory personnel should be done to support the growth of laboratory personnel's professional lives, emphasizing human values and responsibility, and honesty in their work.

Author details

Ashish P. Anjankar[1*], Namrata Anjankar[2] and Vaibhav Anjankar[3]

1 Department of Biochemistry, Jawaharlal Nehru Medical College, Wardha Datta Meghe Institute of Higher Education & Research (Deemed to be University), Wardha, India

2 Department of Clinical Embryology, School of Allied Health Sciences, Datta Meghe Institute of Higher Education & Research (Deemed to be University), Wardha, India

3 Department of Anatomy, Jawaharlal Nehru Medical College, Wardha Datta Meghe Institute of Medical Sciences (Deemed to be University), Wardha, India

*Address all correspondence to: ashish.anjankar@gmail.com

References

[1] Canadian Association of Pathologists. Canadian association of pathologists professionalism and ethics. Available from: http://cap-acp.org/professionalism_and_ethics.cfm. [Last accessed on 2009 Aug 05]

[2] Lock RJ. Rational requesting or rationing testing? Journal of Clinical Pathology. 2004;**57**:121-122

[3] Arora DR, Arora B. Ethics in laboratory medicine. Indian Journal of Medical Microbiology. 2007;**25**:179-180

[4] Burnett L, McQueen MJ, Jonsson JJ, Torricelli F, I.F.C.C. Taskforce on ethics [137]. IFCC position paper: Report of the IFCC taskforce on ethics: Introduction and framework. Clinical Chemistry and Laboratory Medicine. 2007;**45**:1098-1104

[5] ISO 15189:2012 Medical laboratories – requirements for quality and competence. Available from: https://www.iso.org/obp/ui/#iso:std:iso:15189:ed-3:v2:en. [Last accessed on 2016 Jan 09]

[6] AACC. Ethics guidelines. In: Better Health through Laboratory Medicine. Washington, DC, U. S.: American Association of Clinical Chemistry; 11 Sep 2020. Available from: https://www.aacc.org/about-aacc/governance/ethic-guidelines. [Last accessed on 2016 Jan 09]

[7] American Society for Clinical Laboratory Science; Code of Ethics. 2016. Available from: http://www.ascls.org/about-us/code-of-ethics. [Last accessed on 2016 Jan 09]

[8] College of American pathologists principles of ethical and professional conduct. Available from: http://www.cap.org/web/oracle/webcenter/portalapp/pages/searchresults.jspx?searchTerms=cap%20principles%20ethical%20professional&_afrLoo. [Last accessed on 2016 Jan 04]

[9] Pathology Australia code of ethics and practice guidelines. Available from: http://www.pathologyaustralia.com.au/wp-content/uploads/2010/07/02_Pathology-Australia-Code-of-Ethics-and-Practice-Guidelines-November-2012.pdf. [Last Accessed on 2016 Jan 09]

[10] Canadian society for medical laboratory science (SCMLS). Available from: http://www.csmls.org/About-Us/Who-We-Serve/Code-of-Conduct.aspx. [Last Accessed on 2016 Jan 09]

[11] College of Pathologists Pakistan. Ethics for pathologists. Available from: http://www.healthwayslabs.net/docs/ethics.pdf. [Last Accessed on 2016 Jan 09]

[12] Bruns DE, Burtis CA, Gronowski AM, McQueen MJ, Newman A, Jonsson JJ, et al. Variability of ethics education in laboratory medicine training programs: Results of an international survey. Clinica Chimica Acta. 2015;**442**:115-118

[13] Declaration of Geneva. Available from: http://www.wma.net/en/30publications/10policies/g1/wma_declarationofgeneva_A4_EN.pdf. [Last accessed on 2016 Jan 09]

[14] Declaration of Helsinki. Available from: http://www.wma.net/en/30publications/10policies/b3/17c.pdf. [Last accessed on 2016 Jan 09]

[15] Belmont Report. Available from: http://www.hhs.gov/ohrp/

humansubjects/guidance/belmont.html. [Last accessed on 2016 Jan 09]

[16] Allen MJ, Powers ML, Gronowski KS, Gronowski AM. Human tissue ownership and use in research: What laboratorians and researchers should know. Clinical Chemistry. 2010;**56**:1675-1682

[17] Charo RA. Body of research – Ownership and use of human tissue. The New England Journal of Medicine. 2006;**355**:1517-1519

[18] van Diest PJ. No consent should be needed for using leftover body material for scientific purposes for. BMJ. 2002;**325**:648-651

[19] Bathe OF, McGuire AL. The ethical use of existing samples for genome research. Genetics in Medicine. 2009;**11**:712-715

[20] Piva E, Plebani M. Interpretative reports and critical value. Clinica Chimica Acta. 2009;**404**:52-58

[21] Green MJ, Botkin JR. "Genetic exceptionalism" in medicine: Clarifying the differences between genetic and non-genetic tests. Annals of Internal Medicine. 2003;**138**:571-575

Chapter 12

Medical Mistakes – A Romanian Approach

Codrin Horea Rebeleanu and Dana Doroftei

Abstract

In Romania, the medicolegal (forensic) expertise report is created in any case of medical malpractice, at the request of the police, the prosecutor's office, or the court of law. These reports are created for both deceased and alive patients when they or their relatives file a complaint. These forensic medical reports may or may not be taken into consideration by the court of law in the process of each particular trial. In the following chapter, we shall present two cases in which the physicians were accused of malpractice under the Romanian jurisdiction, one in which the court did not take the forensic report into consideration and another case in which, based on the report, the physician was deemed innocent.

Keywords: medical malpractice, medicolegal (forensic) expertise report, Romanian jurisdiction, medical mistakes, medical emergency

1. Introduction

Romania ranks first in the EU in terms of the share of deaths from treatable causes. If at the European level the average of the 27 states is 91 deaths due to treatable causes per 100,000 inhabitants, in Romania the figure is 210 per 100,000 inhabitants [1]. Out of which, a fair share of deaths occurs due to medical mistakes in diagnosis or treatment.

Romania, as a member state of the EU, in accordance with Directive 24/2011 of the European Parliament and the Council, is obliged to own patient protection systems and means of compensation in case of emerging prejudice in medical assistance [2].

Worldwide, there are two options for assessing compensation for patients in case of prejudice: the system based on the mistake/error/negligence of health service providers, which involves taking actions in the court of law, and the system based strictly on compensating patients in case of prejudice (the no-fault system), which does not investigate the culpability of health service providers but only the severity of the prejudice; thus, in the first phase, the courts are not requested to arbitrate these situations. Romania has a mixed system, which is mainly focused on identifying and holding accountable all those who are guilty of the respective prejudice [3].

Although there were projects of implementing a medical malpractice law [4], they were not finalized; the definition of this legal entity is included in Law 95/2006 (which is the fundamental law of healthcare system organization in Romania). Thus,

IntechOpen

art. 653 defines medical malpractice as "the professional error committed in the exercise of the medical act [...], causing damage to the patient, involving the civil liability of the medical staff and the supplier of medical, sanitary, and pharmaceutical products and services" [5].

Medical malpractice is evaluated in Romania by various extrajudicial committees, which, however, cannot determine the amount of compensation to be paid to those prejudiced: the malpractice committee of the college of physician (institution that offers the free practice license to doctors, which can, under certain conditions, suspend or cancel the right to free practice), or the Malpractice Committee of the Directorate of Public Health.

The first committee, when acknowledging the existence of a medical error, has the role of recommending disciplinary sanctioning of the accused doctor, and the second one establishes the guilt or innocence of the medical personnel, but without having the possibility of applying any penalties. Neither of these two committees has the role of establishing the amount of compensation the prejudiced patients.

The compensation of the patients is done either amicably, through negotiation between the accused physician, the insurance company with which he has malpractice insurance and the patient, or judicially, in a criminal or civil trial. Anytime the outcome leads to the court of law, the judge will be able to give a ruling only after a medicolegal expertise report is provided [5].

The forensic medical expertise report is only performed at the request of the police, the prosecutor's office, or the court in case of medical malpractice, regardless of whether the injured patient is alive or deceased. The court may or may not take into account the conclusions of the specialty committees or those of the forensic expertise report [5].

When preparing the forensic medical report, the evaluation of the medical data also involves whether during the diagnostic or therapeutic procedures, the medical guidelines issued for each type of pathology by the Ministry of Health, respectively. The diagnostic and treatment protocols (which represent the adaptation of the guidelines to the particular conditions of each healthcare institution) have been followed accordingly.

According to the Romanian Health Law [6], the healthcare institutions in which prejudice-producing medical acts take place have a civil liability for the damages caused to the patients due to medical mistakes.

The amount of compensation is established by the court and includes the evaluation of material prejudice (additional medical expenses summed with the unacquired income during working incapacity period) and moral prejudice (physical pain, esthetic, juvenile, and sexual prejudice) [7].

To bring further exemplification of the subject, we used sources out of our own medical case history, combined with the information that we identified on the website of the Ministry of Justice regarding the evolution of these cases. Only cases that have been finalized from a judicial point of view and are closed for more than 5 years ago have been used. The cases have been rendered anonymous.

2. Case presentation

2.1 Case number 1

Criminal Law Decision no. xxxx/2015 of the court of appeal:

On November 172006, a 5-year-old girl was admitted to a city hospital for a productive cough that started 12 hours before coming to the hospital; pediatrician X injected her with an amp of ampicillin, 5 minutes later the child went into cardiorespiratory arrest.

The patient presents unsatisfactory response to the resuscitation maneuvers in the first 15 minutes, thus being transferred to a specialized university clinic, having the following referral diagnosis: "1. Cardiorespiratory failure. 2. Cardio-respiratory arrest. 3. Pulmonary edema. 4. Cerebral edema. 5. Coma gr. II." She was intubated for 2 days, then the following therapeutic plan was established and given to the patient:

The therapeutic plan had the following objectives:

- Ensuring adequate respiratory function (aspiration of secretions, aerosol therapy with ACC, administration of mucolytics-expectorants, change of position, tapping, anti-infective treatment, and oxygen therapy in case of need) and maintenance of metabolic balance through parenteral nutrition and nutrition *via* nasogastric tube.

- Anti-infective treatment using multiple antibiotic therapies (2–3 antibiotics), antimycotic, and iv gamma-globulin. The antibiogram for *Klebsiella pneumoniae* as well as that for *Pyocyanin (pseudomonas aeruginosa bacterium)* (both multiresistant germs) required the introduction of ciprofloxacin in the therapeutic plan as well.

- Control of the cerebral edema, Neuro-roborant (restorative) therapy, muscle relaxants, and anticonvulsants.

- Physiotherapy, hepatoprotective and cholestasis treatment, stress ulcer prevention, antithermic measures, central venous catheter heparinization, and anemia treatment.

The evolution was undulating with periods of improvement (improvement of coma and control of infection) alternating with periods of aggravation (clinical-biological signs of serious infection, marked agitation, and convulsions). She presented allergic-type manifestations during treatment with ciprofloxacin (which was discontinued) and the picture of an anaphylactic shock at the first administration of ampicillin.

After receiving medical care, during repeated hospitalizations, for over 4 months, she was discharged from the hospital with the following diagnosis: "Deafferentation syndrome with decerebration outline, spastic tetraplegia, post CPR status, anaphylactic shock to ampicillin. Left vocal cord paralysis. Bronchopneumonia with pseudomonas aeruginosa, klebsiella and enterobacter. Grade II respiratory insufficiency. Drug-induced toxic hepatitis. Acute rotavirus enterocolitis. Mycotic stomatitis. Deficient and intra-infectious anemia, Weight hypotrophy."

The opinion of the Malpractice Committee of the County Medical College was requested, which, by decision no. x/2007, has established the following:

Following the deliberations, the following aspects were retained:

1. The initial clinical diagnosis: Acute bronchopneumonia and acute respiratory failure were established correctly and later confirmed (Children's Emergency Clinical Hospital).

2. The therapeutic attitude was appropriate to the presumptive clinical diagnosis, by associating anti-inflammatory, antispasmodic, steroid medication with a first-line antibiotic—ampicillin—which the patient received repeatedly for recurrent respiratory infections.

3. The intravenous route of administration is a usual practice in pediatrics, and the combination of hydrocortisone hemisuccinate and ampicillin is allowed intravenously.

4. The alleged anaphylactic shock caused by ampicillin cannot be proven, and the prolonged apnea may have originated from the strong productive cough with viscous tracheobronchial secretions; the previous good tolerance to ampicillin, tested in the previous administrations of this antibiotic to the patient, was taken into account.

5. The cardiorespiratory resuscitation maneuvers performed immediately by the medical staff of the pediatric department and continued by the anesthesiologist, led to the recovery of cardiac functions and spontaneous breathing; the prolonged apnea time caused the remaining clinical picture: Deafferentation syndrome with decerebration outline. Spastic quadriplegia after resuscitated cardiorespiratory arrest: The duration of effective cardiorespiratory resuscitation was determined by the location of the pediatric and intensive care wards on different floors, within the city hospital.

6. Dr. X, pediatrician did not commit medical errors.

This opinion was challenged, requesting the opinion of the Higher (National) Discipline Committee of the College of physicians:

By recording all existing medical data, in this case, the college of physicians considered the diagnostic attitude to be appropriate, the clinical (fever, hyper-leukocytosis >20,000 1/m, neutrophilia 81 %) and biological symptomatology justifying the presumption of bacterial respiratory infection and consequently the administration of treatment based on antibacterial antibiotics.

The anamnestic data specify the previous use of ampicillin, without adverse reactions, the intracutaneous testing of ampicillin not being indicated in this case—in accordance with the therapeutic guidelines. As for the diagnosis of respiratory and cardiac syncope through viscous bronchopulmonary secretions, this is less likely in a preschool girl, being much more likely that of anaphylactic shock.

The veracity of this diagnosis, difficult or impossible to verify through clinical explorations, was proven by the repetition of the anaphylactic accident induced by ampicillin in February 2007.

Regarding the therapeutic attitude, considering the clinical symptoms described (fever, cough, dyspnea, and pulmonary rales) in the conditions of hyper-leukocytosis and neutrophilia, the administration of treatment with ampicillin was a correct measure.

Regardless of the presumed diagnosis, the cause of the cardiorespiratory syncope, the therapeutic measures used (PEV—hydrosaline, airway clearance, administration of adrenaline and hydrocortisone hemisuccinate followed by assisted ventilation, cardiac massage, etc.) were adequate. The promptness of the resuscitation maneuvers and the therapeutic attitude throughout the hospitalization were correctly adapted to the clinical status of the patient.

The following are concluded:

1. Anaphylactic reactions to drugs represent very rare iatrogenic events (below 0.01 % of all ampicillin administrations).

2. The allergenic risk of antibiotics from the penicillin and cephalosporin groups is known, but these reactions are unpredictable, with cases of anaphylactic shock to ampicillin being described in the literature even without known previous exposure and side effects.

3. The patient is known with previous exposure to ampicillin, without adverse reactions and without presenting any risk factors—atopy or previous allergic manifestations.

4. To establish the diagnosis of anaphylactic risk to ampicillin, unfortunately, there are no specific screening methods, and the ampicillin cutaneous test is not recommended for people without suspicion of allergy to penicillin-type antibiotics, as it lacks diagnostic relevance.

5. In the present case, the intensity of the anaphylactic reaction was particularly high, considering the absence of any clinical attenuation that was supposed to appear due to simultaneous administration of hydrocortisone hemisuccinate with ampicillin.

The Higher Disciplinary Committee concludes that the facts and circumstances did not constitute a deviation from good medical practice and decides. According to art. 26 and art. 31, chapter III of the regulation on the organization and development of the activities of the disciplinary committees to reject the appeal and uphold decision no. x/2007 dated 05.11.2007 issued by the local disciplinary committee of the County College of Physicians.

The official medicolegal report records all medical data and concludes that:

The committee assesses the case of the minor, as a case of anaphylactic shock to ampicillin, of very high intensity, in a person who did not present in her personal history an atopic terrain or allergic manifestations, without being able to completely exclude a respiratory and cardiac syncope through aspiration of viscous bronchopulmonary secretions. We appreciate that both the diagnostic and therapeutic attitudes, in this case, were in accordance with the level of current medical knowledge, without being able to conclude a deficiency in the provision of medical care attributable to the doctor.

The patient's parents also hired a private forensic expert, who prepared an expert opinion, by which he sustained the medical fault by stating that the doctor is guilty of not performing an ampicillin cutaneous test.

Since there are two forensic expertise reports with divergent conclusions, a report of new forensic expertise is requested to be made by the Higher Commission within INML-Bucharest. In the conclusions formulated, INML Bucharest states that there are no errors committed by Dr. X, given that the cutaneous test for ampicillin is not recommended, being devoid of diagnostic relevance.

Disregarding the forensic conclusions and the ones elaborated by the Disciplinary Committee of the College of Physicians, the court of appeal sentences the doctor to pay the civil parties the following amounts:

- To the civil side Y. The sum of 100,000 euros as moral damages, the amount of 3000 lei as a monthly annuity from 17.11. 2006 to 02.04.2014, and the amount of 2916 lei as monthly life annuity from 02.04.2014 until the physical and mental infirmity ceases.

- To the civil parties Z. and W. The sum of 96,000 lei as civil compensation for material damages and the sum of 50,000 euros each as civil compensation for moral damages.

- To the civil side V in the amount of 2106 lei monthly starting from 04/30/2007, in the amount of 1206 lei from 05/07/2007 as civil compensation for material damages consisting of unrealized income.

Regarding the penal aspect of the trial, the court considered that as far as this head of accusation is concerned, the case cannot be judged due to the occurrence of the statute of limitation (prescription).

2.2 Case number 2

On November 13, 2016, at 12:10 am, a 63-year-old man was hospitalized urgently for retrosternal pain and anxiety, the clinical symptoms starting 3 hours before presentation to the emergency room; the diagnosis recorded in the medical records is acute myocardial infarction (the electrocardiogram performed shows ST-segment elevation in V1-V5).

The patient's condition and monitored parameters improve during hospitalization in response to the treatment administered. At 2:30 p.m., the patient presents cardio-respiratory arrest—cardiorespiratory resuscitation maneuvers are performed without success, and the patient is declared dead at 3:20 p.m.

During hospitalization, the request to transfer the patient to the Cardiology Department of the Cluj-Napoca Heart Institute is accepted, a transfer that cannot be carried out due to the lack of authorized medical personnel to transport him by ambulance and the impossibility of using a helicopter due to unfavorable weather conditions.

According to the medical protocols, conventional treatment is administered, which includes:

- Sodium heparin—5000 units;

- Plavix 75 mg 8 tablets;

- Aspenter one 75 mg tablet;

- Mialgin—3 ml of 2 ml dilution plus 8 ml physiological serum;

- Nitronal—3 vials (30 ml with 20 ml physiological serum) were administered by injectomat 1 ml/hour;

- Atacand of 8 mg one tablet;

- Simvastatin of 10 mg one tablet.

The patient stabilizes after the administration of the medication, but later at 2:30 p.m., he suffers a cardiorespiratory arrest for which cardiopulmonary resuscitation is performed. According to the existent medical protocols, cardiorespiratory resuscitation maneuvers are performed by administering adrenaline 14 ampoules, cordarone 2 ampoules and an electric shock, plus cardiac massage, manual ventilation, and oxygen therapy.

Thrombolytic drugs, such as reteplase and streptokinase, were not available in the emergency room at the present hospital.

The treatment applied at presentation is stipulated in the acute myocardial infarction treatment protocol and was administered with the approval of the cardiologist from the Cluj-Napoca Heart Institute.

From the address issued by the hospital, we assess the following statements:

The city hospital does not have a department for emergency admissions, and the emergencies are organized and admitted by the emergency room system. There is no emergency physician, and the emergency room nightshifts are provided by doctors from other specialties that are available in the hospital (internists, gastroenterologists, and neurologists), which have no competence in the administration of thrombolytic drugs. There is no corresponding equipment to supervise the thrombolytic treatment.

There were no thrombolytic drugs at the hospital pharmacy either before or on 11/13/2016.

Order 1706/2007 regarding the management and organization of emergency reception units and departments, in art. 37 and 39, explicitly states that category IV hospitals (the city hospital is a category IV-a hospital) that do not have emergency departments due to lack of human or material resources will organize the reception of emergencies in the emergency room system.

In the event that the hospital cannot provide the definitive treatment through thrombolysis, it has the obligation to organize the transfer of the patient, in the shortest possible time, to a hospital with a higher level of competence, which has the ability to apply the definitive treatment, usually a regional hospital or at least one that is registered as a competence level II hospital (art. 1.8 and art. 7 of the Order of the Ministry of Health no. 1764/2006).

In the event that the patient requires transfer to another health unit, the doctor on call organizes the transfer in accordance with the existent legal provisions. The transfer decision is taken by the doctor on call together with the doctors on call from the health unit to which the respective patient is to be transferred.

In this case, contact was made with the on-call doctor from the cardiology department of the Cluj-Napoca Heart Institute in order to transfer the patient with acute myocardial infarction under medical supervision (a certain kind of ambulance was requested, with the necessity of having a physician on board due to the current status of the patient) receiving the acceptance for the transport, but the transfer was not carried out, due the lack of specialized medical personnel necessary.

Furthermore, due to the fact that the physician requested was already carrying out another emergency transport, another physician was requested from home to carry out the transfer either to Cluj-Napoca or to the Bistrita County Hospital, which has an emergency reception unit and a cardiology department where the thrombolytic treatment and necessary specialized physicians are available. The transfer did not take place due to the impossibility of transport, and the patient died two hours from the presentation in the emergency room.

The order of the Ministry of Health mentioned above also specifies in letter "E" point 35, for emergency department type 1 and 2 the mandatory existence of thrombolytic medication, although for the emergency reception room these can be mandatory or not (+/–). For the emergency room system (also existent at the hospital in which the patient was admitted), the mandatory existence is not stipulated for this medication.

Following the evaluation of the medical data from the present file, as well as the additional documents requested by the members of the hospital's committee, the following answers are stated:

1. Based on the medical documents and the actions of the medical personnel, it cannot be established with accuracy whether the patient's death could have been prevented in the case of transfer to another hospital unit, with superior equipment.

2. According to the medical report issued by the Cardiology Department-County Hospital, the doctor on call requested the transfer of the patient according to the protocol provided for the situation of acute myocardial infarction type STEMI.

3. The medical treatment administered to the patient at the city hospital, from the time of admission until death, was adequate to the symptoms, diagnosis, and equipment owned by the hospital.

4. We consider that in the case of a patient who suffered an acute myocardial infarction, myocardial revascularization (invasive or medicinal; we specify that none of the methods were available in the hospital) was indicated. We cannot say whether the patient would have survived if such an intervention had been applied.

5. In the patient's medical situation, we consider that transport to another hospital unit, with superior equipment, was indicated. We cannot establish whether the patient would have survived a transport to the Heart Institute in Cluj-Napoca.

The conclusions of the autopsy are as follows:
Macroscopic anatomic-pathological diagnosis:

- Myocardial and coronary sclerosis. Aortic atherosclerosis. Acute myocardial infarction.

- Hepatic steatosis.

- Congested viscera (stasis).

The histopathological exam confirmed the autopsy findings.

a. The death of the patient was nonviolent.

b. It was due to acute cardiocirculatory failure caused by an acute myocardial infarction.

c. Death may date from November 13, 2016.

According to the medical report issued by the Cardiology Department-County Hospital, the medical treatment administered to the patient at the city hospital, from the time of admission until death, was adequate to the symptoms, diagnosis, and equipment of the hospital.

"We consider that in the case of the patient who suffered an acute myocardial infarction, myocardial revascularization (invasive or medicinal; we specify that none of the methods were available in the hospital in question) was indicated. We cannot say whether the patient would have survived if such an intervention had been applied."

"In the patient's medical situation, we consider that the transport to another hospital unit, with superior equipment, was indicated. We cannot establish whether the patient would have survived a transport to the Heart Institute in Cluj-Napoca."

The prosecutor's office found that there was no fault on the part of the doctor, closing the case. The solution was not contested.

3. Conclusions

1. In Romania, medical malpractice can be filed in different forums, with different results, as follows:

   - For the simple ascertaining of malpractice, without any other consequences (with the exception of the situation where they are self-assumed by the doctor and assumed by the insurance company with which the respective doctor has malpractice insurance), there is the Malpractice Committee of the Directorate of Public health.

   - For the disciplinary sanction of the physician in the context in which he deviated from the legal provisions, there is the Disciplinary Committee of the College of Physicians.

   - In order to establish the guilt in the court of law, this having criminal and civil consequences, there is the possibility that the injured patient or the deceased patient's relatives should address the police, the prosecutor's office, or directly the court of law, in which case the forensic expertise report is mandatory. In this situation, apart from the official forensic expertise report, any of the parties can hire a private forensic expert, who will compile an expert opinion.

2. The court may take into account any of the conclusions of the committees or the forensic expertise reports or may disregard them when a sentence is established. This is one of the reasons why Romania pays large sums of money to people who were initially convicted and who challenged the sentences at the European Court of Human Rights.

3. In the presented cases, we assess both of these situations in which the court did or did not take into consideration the forensic medical reports created for the case. Regarding the multiple malpractice complaints filed in Romania, these reports have a major importance in determining the guilt of the physician, changing the outcome of the trial and serving as supportive measures in concluding these cases.

Conflict of interest

The authors declare no conflict of interest.

Abbreviations

EU	European Union
INML	The National Institute of Legal Medicine.
STEMI	ST-elevation myocardial infarction

Appendix

In Romania, the medical emergency ward system is divided by the extension and medical personnel it has—an emergency department is a more extensive unit that benefits from more specialized physicians while an emergency room is a smaller, emergency reception unit (which, like in the cases presented, does not have access to certain medication or specialized physicians in this domain).

Author details

Codrin Horea Rebeleanu[1*] and Dana Doroftei[2]

1 University of Medicine and Pharmacy "Iuliu Hațieganu" Cluj Napoca, Romania

2 University of Medicine, Pharmacy, Science and Technology "George Emil Palade" Târgu Mureș, Romania

*Address all correspondence to: soupdotcom@gmail.com

References

[1] State of Health in the EU—Romania—Country Health Profile 2021. Available from: https://www.oecd.org/publications/romania-country-health-profile-2021-74ad9999-en.htm. [Accessed: December 13, 2021]

[2] Directive 2011/24/EU of the European Parliament and of the Council of 9 March 2011 on the application of patients' rights in cross-border. Available from: https://eur-lex.europa.eu/legal-content/RO/TXT/?uri=celex%3A32011L0024

[3] Medicina sub asediu? Impactul reclamatiilor privind raspunderea profesionala medicala, Bianca Hanganu, Beatrice Gabriela Ioan, Iasi, Editura Gr. T. Popa. 2022. ISBN 978-606-544-730-1

[4] Study on the compensation system for injured patients applicable in Romania. A critical analysis of the draft law on civil liability of medical staff and suppliers (Study on Compensation System for Injured Patients Applicable in Romania. A Critical Analysis of the Draft Law on Civil Liability of Medical Staff and Suppliers), Galați, Sodalitas Publishing House, ISBN 978-606-93503-3-1. Available from: https://papers.ssrn.com/sol3/papers.cfm?abstract_id=2908070

[5] Law no. 271/2004 regarding the approval of Government Ordinance no. 57/2001 for the amendment and completion of Government Ordinance no. 1/2000 regarding the organization of the activity and the functioning of legal medicine institutions. Available from: https://lege5.ro/Gratuit/gu3dqnrr/legea-nr-271-2004-privind-aprobarea-ordonantei-guvernului-nr-57-2001-pentru-modificarea-si-completarea-ordonantei-guvernului-nr-1-2000-privind-organizarea-activitatii-si-functionarea-institutiilor-de-

[6] Law 95/2006, art 655-657. Available from: https://legislatie.just.ro/Public/DetaliiDocument/71139

[7] Malpraxisul medical: particularitatile raspunderii civile medicale: jurisprudenta interna relevanta: malpraxisul profesiilor liberale, Nasui Gabriel Adrian, Bucuresti, Editura Universul Juridic. 2016. ISBN 978-606-673-873-6